Communication Skills for Foreign and Mobile Medical Professionals

Kris Van de Poel · Eddy Vanagt
Ulrike Schrimpf · Jessica Gasiorek

Communication Skills for Foreign and Mobile Medical Professionals

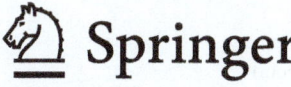

Kris Van de Poel
University of Antwerp
Department of Linguistics
Antwerp
Belgium

North-West University
School of Languages
Potchefstroom
South Africa

Eddy Vanagt
formerly ZNA
Hospital Network Antwerp
Antwerp
Belgium

Ulrike Schrimpf
Charité Berlin
Charité International Academy
Berlin
Germany

Jessica Gasiorek
University of California
Department of Communication
Santa Barbara
California
USA

ISBN 978-3-642-35111-2   ISBN 978-3-642-35112-9   (eBook)
DOI 10.1007/978-3-642-35112-9
Springer Heidelberg New York Dordrecht London

Library of Congress Control Number: 2013936262

Springer is part of Springer Science+Business Media (www.springer.com)

This book is dedicated to the many anonymous trainers in the field who cannot help but communicate with their interns. This book is also dedicated to young 'foreign' doctors such as Bruno, Homa and Chris who, despite all odds, have made the global medical world their home.

Preface

Communication Skills for Foreign and Mobile Medical Professionals (or in short *Medical Communication Skills*) is an evidence-based communication resource book aimed at second language or language-discordant medical professionals, defined as doctors who work in foreign countries, cultures and languages, who are interested in improving or enhancing their communication with both patients and colleagues.

Good doctor–patient communication correlates directly with improved patient health outcomes. Culturally and linguistically appropriate communicative competence is a key skill for medical professionals: it can literally be life-saving.

Given the growing number of mobile medical professionals around the world and the importance of good communication to both patient outcomes and the medical professionals' own professional success, this state-of-the-art resource book is highly relevant. Professionals ranging from senior nursing staff, hospital doctors, interns, general practitioners and heads of department in multilingual or intercultural contexts to human resource managers, language trainers and cultural mediators will all have something to learn from this book.

This is a practitioners' manual for the lower/upper undergraduate, graduate and professional/practitioner levels. It covers the areas of communication skills, effective medical communication, intercultural professional communication, doctor–patient communication and patient-oriented medicine.

This book targets language-discordant medical professionals, a readership that is not served by any book on medical communication currently on the market. The book provides direct answers to the practical needs of the clinical context and can be used for training and teaching purposes both in contact teaching and autonomously. The proposed advice raises the professional's awareness of important issues in face-to-face interaction. *Medical Communication Skills* is the foundation of a medical performance support system containing strategies and tips, examples and short excerpts from intercultural health studies. It offers a wealth of insights into communication structured around the consultation timeline, which all doctors know and have training in.

Medical Communication Skills helps professionals gain insight into doctor–patient communication and is organised around the different phases of any consultation. It emphasises patient-oriented medicine, the ideal style of doctoring in today's Western world. The advice offered shows how communication in general and doctor–patient communication in particular work; where applicable examples are provided. Common misunderstandings between doctors and patients with different cultural/linguistic backgrounds are dealt with specifically and in depth.

Communication in a professional context has a universal basis, and we hope that you, the intended audience, will gain some inspiration and insights from our multifaceted analyses of the topic.

What Can You Expect to Find in This Book

Chapter 1. Interpersonal and Intercultural Communication in Health Care

This chapter outlines the background of the book and introduces terminology and topics vital for understanding interpersonal and intercultural communication in a healthcare context: communication and personal *style*, communication and patient *health outcomes*, *multiculturalism* and cultural *competence* and communication and *mobility*. This book is meant to function as a communication performance support tool. The information in it draws on peer-reviewed, international research and focuses on linguistic and cultural challenges faced by mobile medical professionals.

Chapter 2. The Structure of the Consultation

When patients' physical, mental and social well-being (i.e. the *health triangle*) is not in balance, they may see a doctor. To a consultation, patients bring ideas, concerns and expectations (the *ICE triad*) about health and illness. This triad is situated within a patient's frame of reference and has both individual and cultural characteristics. In the past 30 years, medicine in the Western world has become increasingly *patient-oriented*, and the medical world has adopted a model of the consultation where patient's and doctor's perspectives are given equal weight. In this chapter, we present the *two-perspectives* consultation model, which describes the structure and timeline of the consultation. Structuring a consultation means timing and sequencing five major tasks in a logically ordered way following a mental map (cf. the Calgary-Cambridge Guides): *initiating the session, information gathering, the physical examination, explaining and planning, and closing the session.*

Chapter 3. General Communication Strategies and Skills

In this chapter, we discuss communication skills that can be used across all stages of the consultation. We first focus on how active *listening* skills facilitate, direct and structure interaction with others. Then we explain and illustrate what makes verbal and nonverbal communication appropriate. While the focus of our verbal communication is generally the *content* of our messages, our *attitudes* about what we say are often communicated through our nonverbal communication. The final topic of the chapter is building *rapport*: it helps make both communication and consultations more effective, efficient, supportive and satisfying for both medical professionals and patients.

Chapter 4. Communication Skills Specific to the Consultation

This chapter discusses communication skills and strategies used at specific points during the consultation, providing specific advice for different stages and parts of the consultation. The first part of the consultation begins with an *opening*, followed by *medical history* taking or anamnesis, and concludes with the *physical examination*. Listening is central to these stages. The second half of the consultation focuses on discussion and generally has two components—(1) *explaining* the diagnosis and (2) agreeing on the *management plan*—that follows from this diagnosis. Both successful listening and explaining then allow for a proper *closing* of the session.

Chapter 5. Special Challenges in Medical Communication

During consultations, doctors often have to deal with challenging situations. They can be caused by characteristics of the patients, the content, the communication channel or any combination of these. When *patients* are challenging, clearly structuring the interaction and acknowledging the patient may help. When dealing with sensitive or taboo *topics*, particular care and sensitivity are required. Finally, in telephone and other *mediated consultations*, an explicit and systematic approach to communication can facilitate the conversation. This chapter provides an overview of a range of challenging situations doctors are likely to encounter, and provides strategies to address them.

About the Authors

Eddy Vanagt developed a keen interest in the nature of medical communication during his life as a cardiologist at different hospitals in the Netherlands and Belgium. Over the past 20 years, while supervising and guiding an international group of interns at Antwerp Hospital Network, he compiled strategies and tips from the current literature with the help of feedback from the University of Antwerp's medical skills lab staff and input from project partners in Berlin, Maastricht, Ancona and Gothenburg.

Kris Van de Poel (University of Antwerp—Applied Language Studies and affiliated with North-West University's School for Languages) specialises in curriculum and syllabus design for professional and academic purposes. She developed the resource book's overall format and approach, relying on her teaching and training experience with both foreign and mobile medical professionals and students and her research on this group's needs.

Ulrike Schrimpf while at Charité International Cooperation—Charité International Academy, has co-developed the intercultural component of this book, drawing from years of involvement in teaching, developing and publishing materials for different medical contexts in Germany (*International Doctors, International Nurses, Cross-Cultural Communication*).

Jessica Gasiorek is finalising her doctoral research in the Department of Communication at the University of California, Santa Barbara, studying interpersonal and intergroup communication, focusing on communication accommodation and its consequences across contexts. She is also associated with the University of Antwerp, has collaborated on projects related to this group and has edited the language in this book for an international audience.

All four authors have been collaborating on the European project *Medics on the Move* (2006–2012), for which they carried out research and developed interactive online and mobile communication tools across languages and cultures.

Acknowledgements

Writing a textbook on medical communication skills does not happen overnight and does not happen single-handedly. We have certainly been inspired by the many excellent textbooks on the market. Even though we may not have quoted from them directly, they have paved the way for our better understanding of the intricacies of professional communication in action.

Medical Communication Skills—the running title of this book—couldn't have been realised without the comments and observations of many people who have, knowingly or unknowingly, contributed to this project, but, of course, we remain responsible for the content and format of this book, and any errors or inconsistencies in this text are our own.

We would like to thank sincerely all the medical professionals who over the years have worked with the materials and commented on them, have taken part in the experiments and have interacted with our presentations and publications.

Special thanks go to the participants in the needs analysis: Dr. Tineke Brunfaut, Lancaster University/University of Antwerp, for her analysis of the language data; staff and medical students from Antwerp University Faculty of Medicine and Faculty of Arts; Dean Prof. Dr. Paul Van de Heyning, Faculty of Medicine University of Antwerp; managerial, medical and secretarial staff in the Region Västra Götaland and at the Sahlgrenska Academy, as well as interpreters at Tolkcentralen in Göteborg; staff and medical students from Charité Hochschulmedizin Berlin; language staff at Folkuniversitetet Göteborg; Dr. Peter Lyndrup from Aabenraa Sygehus and Dr. David Dynnes Ørsted Herlev Sygehus, of Antwerp Hospital Network zna; Dr. Chris Boon, emergency physician and surgeon; Dr. Katrien Bervoets, internist-intensivist; Dr. Jean-Paul Alexander, anaesthetist-intensivist; Dr. Philippe Vandenberghe, paediatric cardiologist; Dr. Juliarto Bunarto, cardiac surgeon; Dr. Wesseling, gynaecologist-obstetrician; Prof. Dr. Med. Markus Nöthen, human genetics; and Prof. Dr. Sven Cichon, genetic counsellor, at the University of Bonn; of Azienda Ospedaliera Umberto I, Ospedali Riuniti of Ancona: Dr. Roberto Penna, Dr. Alfio Ulissi, Dr. Andrea Soccetti, and Dr. Mahoud Yehia; of Charité Hochschulmedizin Berlin: Dr. Evjenia Toubekis, Dr. Caroline Guthke, and Dr. Philipp Knape; staff from the Health Department and the Institute of Communication and Health of the Scuola Universitaria Professionale della Svizzera Italiana (SUPSI); Dr. Luc Debaene and Dr. Katrien Bombeke from the Communication skills lab at the University of Antwerp; the training staff of the skills lab at Charité International Cooperation and

Charité International Academy; and Prof. Göran Bonders from the Nordic School for Public Health and President of the Sahlgrenska Academy in Gothenburg.

We also thank the many doctors-testees and in particular: Dr. Francesco Agostoni, Dr. Chris Boone, Fiona Boone-Haworth and Dr. Frank Van den Brande from the Hospital Network Antwerp; Dr. Annett Buettner, Dr. Julia Flor, Dr. Degaulle Najm, Dr. Svetlana Najm and Dr. Arya Payvand from Västra Götalandsregionen; Dr. Jerzy Gesla and Dr. Dmitriy Shilenok from Kolding Sygehus and Dr. Mirek Ziolkiewicz, Aabenraa Sygehus; Dr. Homa Hosseini from the University Hospital Antwerp; Dr. Bruno Schwagten from Rotterdam University Hospital; and Dr. Ward Vanagt and Dr. Veronique Moulaert from Maastricht University.

We would like wholeheartedly to acknowledge the *Medics on the Move* (*MoM*) project partners for actively and creatively engaging in the topic of medical communication and for their inspirational support:

Randi Myhre from Immigrant-institutet Borås; Kylene De Angelis from Training 2000 Mondavio; Ine De Rycke from Universiteit Antwerpen; Ulla Ekström from Västra Götalandsregionen Vänersborg; Christina Eriksson and Camilla Johansson from Immigrant-institutet Borås and Folkuniversitetet Göteborg; Thomas Hutchins from TeAM Hutchins AB Sollebrunn; Tove Nygaard Knudsen from Videnscenter for Integration; Arne Oehlsen from Charité International Cooperation; Lene Rybner from Videnscenter for Integration and Dr. Elena Tomassini from S.S.M.L Fondazione Universitaria San Pellegrino.

Special thanks go to Dr. Nataliya Berbyuk Lindström from Immigrant-institutet Borås and Chalmers University of Technology Gothenburg for her input on the intercultural component.

The *MoM* project was made possible by an initial grant of the European Commission—Leonardo da Vinci and started off our search for transcultural medical communication support.

We also want to thank the participants in the master's course Curriculum and Syllabus Design 2007–2008, 2008–2009, 2010–2011 and 2011–2012 for contributing to the discussion on the communication needs of medical professionals and all the international medical students (from EMSA (European Medical Students' Association) and other organisations) who took part in classes prior to going abroad or upon arrival in their new work environment.

Last but not least, thanks to our support networks who have proven very useful and necessary.

Eddy Vanagt
Kris Van de Poel
Ulrike Schrimpf
Jessica Gasiorek

Contents

Interpersonal and Intercultural Communication in Health Care

1

Contents

K. Van de Poel et al., *Communication Skills for Foreign and Mobile Medical Professionals,*
DOI 10.1007/978-3-642-35112-9_1, © Springer-Verlag Berlin Heidelberg 2013

This chapter primarily introduces:

- The nature of communication in a clinical setting
- Why appropriate medical communication matters

Moreover, it highlights:

- What the book *Medical Communication Skills* stands for
- Why *Medical Communication Skills* is a reference manual
- What you will get out of it
- The best way to use it

The overall aim and objective of this book is to raise your awareness about medical communication and we hope that this chapter contains the first steps.

1.1   Medical Communication Skills

1.1.1   Communication in a Clinical Setting

Medical Communication Skills is a resource book offering insights in how communication in a medical context is shaped. Medical professionals communicate in different **clinical settings,** including:

- Consultations
- Examinations
- Handoffs
- Meetings

They also communicate in different **constellations**, including contact with:

- Patients
- Patients' relatives
- Colleagues
- Administrators

This book focuses on doctor–patient communication during the consultation, because the consultation is the basic doctor–patient encounter. Consultations in medicine occur in widely different contexts, from new to follow-up appointments, emergencies to routine check-ups and in locations from consultation room to bedside. Although it may at first seem that there are many differences between communicating in each of these diverse settings, the overall objectives and skills required are remarkably consistent. The basic communication skills needed to navigate these situations not only are the same in these different consultation settings but apply equally beyond the consultation, during corridor meetings, staff meetings and informal discussions over tea or coffee.

1.1.2   *Medical Communication Skills*: A Reference Book

In this first chapter, we want to introduce some terms and concepts which are essential to better understand the world of medical communication. Since *Medical Communication Skills* really is a reference manual, we have tried not to make this introductory chapter too long or too academic in nature. If you would like more background on the nature of communication more generally, any introductory book on communication, pragmatics or intercultural management will be a good reference. We have provided recommendations for additional reading and background on issues specific to intercultural and/or medical communication at the end of each chapter (all but one in English).

Since time is precious in all professional contexts, but specifically in clinical settings, we expect that very few of you will read this book from cover to cover. We have therefore designed this manual a reference book, so you can easily access what you need, when you need it. The information in this book draws on peer-reviewed, international research; our goal is to present it to you in clear, accessible language, so you can benefit from what communication and applied linguistics scholars know about medical communication without having to go through the literature yourself.

1.1.3   The Book's Foundations

1.1.3.1 Patient-Oriented Medicine

The book emphasises patient-oriented medicine, which is widely considered the *ideal* style of doctoring in today's Western world. As mentioned above, it is grounded in a critical reading of the international literature on doctor–patient interaction. This work is evidence-based and draws on years of experience engaging with aspiring doctors of different nationalities and helping and training them to communicate more efficiently and effectively and becoming the doctors their patients wish for.

1.1.3.2 The Book's History: A Performance Support Tool

This book was conceived in the framework of the European project *Medics on the Move—Language Solutions for Mobile Medical Professionals*, a performance support tool in six languages for international and mobile medical professionals (www.medicsmove.eu). The tips offered in the *Medics on the Move* doctor–patient scenarios were compiled in its *Communication Manual*, which provided insights into how communication works both in general and in doctor–patient interactions. The *manual* was reviewed by different European skills labs to ensure its applicability and usability across countries and communities, and it benefited tremendously from these discussions.

In the second phase of the project, the manual was extended with **intercultural** reflections drawing on the extensive literature on the topic. This version of the manual was after-end project rewritten and extended to create a stand-alone reference book—this book.

1.1.3.3 The Book's Challenges and Intended Audience

In *Medical Communication Skills*, we will introduce **general communication topics** and challenges to the context of mobile medical professionals. Since mobility among medical professionals is on the increase (European Commission 2011; OECD 2008), it requires that doctors be able to provide culturally competent care to patients of different cultural backgrounds. This means that doctors and other health-care staff need to be knowledgeable and skilful intercultural communicators. Sometimes, problems in intercultural consultations can be the result of misunderstandings related to the cultural differences between doctor and patient. Although health-care staff are doing their best, there are many outside factors that can influence patients' behaviour and trust in doctors, including migration stress, discrimination and the patient's economic and social situation.

Through this book, we hope to make you (more) aware of what to look and listen for in intercultural consultations, so that you can avoid misunderstandings and communicate productively and positively with your patients.

1.2   Communication in Health Care

1.2.1   Communication and Personal Style

Much of *how* we communicate is automatic and **unconscious**. In most situations, we do not actively think about what we are doing. However, we have a certain sense of what sounds and feels right; we also each have preferences in our language use. When speaking a foreign language, we also have idiosyncrasies; sometimes, we may use outdated or 'fossilised' forms, or not know a particular jargon, style or tone well enough to use it for professional purposes. These issues with language may cause tension and/or problems in professional interactions, particularly with people we are not familiar with. This resource book aims to make you more **aware** of your own communication style and help you adapt it to your professional needs.

1.2.2   Communication and Patient Health Outcomes

Communication in a medical context is built on trust between medical professional and patient. Patients coming to see a doctor are vulnerable and may be emotional: needing medical care often leaves people worried, angry and/or confused. This is the person you have to communicate with and for whom you have to adapt your communication.

Research has shown that a more patient-centred communication results in a more effective consultation for both patient and doctor. Research has also shown a direct correlation between effective patient-centred communication and patient health outcomes (Stewart 1995; Travaline et al. 2005). Good communication facilitates achieving all the goals of the medical encounter, including accuracy and effectiveness of planning and management, efficiency and time management, collaboration on management plans and satisfaction for both patient and doctor.

However, the question remains: *what is good communication?* As a start, actively listening to the patient's needs, wants, desires, ideas, concerns and expectations is a crucial component and a skill which can be learned (see Chap. 2), then it is imperative to harmonise verbal and nonverbal communication (see Chap. 3) and consistently focusing on these skills in every component of the consultation (see Chap. 4), even when the partners, content or channel of communication are challenging (see Chap. 5).

Not only does the quality of doctor–patient communication directly influence the quality of patient care, but also the quality of your communication with colleagues has an effect on health outcomes (e.g. Gasiorek and Van de Poel 2012; Gesensway 2006; Hewett et al. 2009; Watson et al. 2012). However, linguistic and cultural training for most mobile medical professionals (and indeed doctors more generally) in Western Europe is minimal. Medical communication support guides (such as the Calgary-Cambridge guides for the medical interview by Silverman et al. (2006) and Kurtz et al. (2006) but also the different guides to physical examination and history taking by the group around Bickley (Bickley 2007; Bickley and Szilagiy 2007; Prabhu and Bickley 2007) or communication handbooks like Tate 2007 and Pendleton et al. 2007) generally target native speakers rather than language learners, and typically mention the use of a foreign language as just one of many issues in cross-cultural communication without providing any solutions or prescriptions to address ensuing communication problems.

1.2.3   A Question of Language or Culture

1.2.3.1   Language, Culture, Race and Ethnicity

There is consistent evidence that not only language but also culture, race and ethnicity have a substantial influence on the quality of the doctor–patient relationship (Ferguson and Candib 2002; Berbyuk Lindström 2008).

According to research on foreign language communication in medical contexts, the nature of the potential communication issues is diverse. **Linguistically**, foreign doctors may experience different problems, like, for instance:

- Understanding regional and colloquial language
- Using colloquial speech and common medical language
- Using medical vocabulary, brand names and abbreviations
- Understanding and using nonverbal communication (such as appropriate levels of eye contact)
- Providing appropriate emotional support, including expressing care and concern
- Giving and accepting feedback (e.g. Fitzgerald 2003; Hall et al. 2004; Pilotto et al. 2007)

Culturally, foreign doctors may lack knowledge that is relevant to the health-care domain and/or follow different norms or standards for consultation and treatment (e.g. Fiscella and Frankel 2000; Lockyer et al. 2007; McMahon 2004). Underlying to this all, foreign medical professionals may also fear discrimination or mistreatment on the basis of cultural differences (e.g. Fiscella and Frankel 2000; Moore and Rhodenbaugh 2002).

All in all, the majority of misunderstandings between doctors and patients with a different cultural background can be attributed to the following domains:

- The expectations of the clinical encounter
- Verbal as well as nonverbal communication patterns

Deficiencies in verbal communication patterns seem to be easier to identify. However, in a mobile world, bridging language and cultural barriers between physicians and patients requires a holistic approach (Hall et al. 2004; Hornberger et al. 1996, 1997; Lu and Corbett 2012).

Before we move to the linguistic barriers which doctors and patients encounter, we will first explain how we understand 'culture'.

1.2.3.2 Culture Versus Cultures

This book wants to stress that there is no single culture for a given country, but rather that people's preferences, norms and expectation for communication come from a blend of individual or personal styles and cultures of regions. The concept of 'culture' is dynamic and comprises a learned set of beliefs, values, norms and social practices shared by a group of people (see Schouten and Meeuwesen 2006 for a review of the literature):

- **Beliefs** refer to the basic understanding of a group of people about what the world is like or what is true or false.
- **Values** refer to what a group of people defines as good and bad and what it regards as important.
- **Norms** refer to rules for appropriate behaviour in concordance with the beliefs and values. It includes expectations people have of one another and of themselves.
- **Social practices** are the cultural component of the predictable behaviour patterns that members of a culture typically follow.

While people from a country do share sets of beliefs, values, norms and social practices, not everyone will match the stereotypes of the national culture(s) they belong to. A French woman could share the same beliefs as an Arab man because she has converted to Islam; a German who has been living in Scandinavia for 5 years could share some of the basic common values with his host culture. Thus, rather than just determining where someone is from and making assumptions, it is important to find out which beliefs, values, norms and social practices are important to that person. Only when we understand this can we communicate in a proper, effective way with this person.

1.2.3.3 Stereotyping

When we try to grasp the essence of a foreign culture, we often end up using stereotypes. Stereotypes are conventional, formulaic and oversimplified generalisations of a culture, person or situation. A lot of jokes are, for example, built around the notion that Italians are talkative, Swedes are reserved and cold, Germans are efficient, Americans are informal and Finns are silent. However, jokes and generalisations do not take into account that people have personalities and that their individual character plays an important role in communication.

If doctors do not explore patients' beliefs and views of their own symptoms and illness, they risk making assumptions and stereotyping patients. This can lead not only to conflict, but also to inaccuracy in diagnosis, and to inappropriate treatment, compromising patients' health.

1.2.3.4 Multiculturalism, Intercultural Communication and (Trans) cultural Competence

The concepts of culture and communication have given rise to some interesting and relatively new concepts, such as *multicultural, intercultural* and *transcultural communication and competence*. While all these terms address people with different cultural and linguistic backgrounds, each is slightly different.

The term **multicultural**—which was commonly used to describe American society as consisting of people with different cultural and linguistic backgrounds—highlights the belief that people have the right to conserve their cultural identity, particularly when they are in a new place with different, other cultures. This is now regarded as a rather restrictive view of cultural interaction and contact. The term **intercultural** is frequently used by researchers to describe the interactions between people with different cultural and linguistic backgrounds. Finally, **transcultural** competence (also known as **cultural and linguistic competence** outside of a European context) is a more scientific term which claims that there is no such thing as a 'culture of its own' since the contemporary structure of cultures goes across traditional borders, hence 'transcultural'.

Transcultural Care
Already in the 1940s, Madeleine Leininger, a progressive nurse, realised that recurrent behavioural patterns and needs in children had a cultural basis. Leininger identified a lack of cultural and care knowledge as the missing link to nurses' understanding of patients' beliefs and needs and promoted the universal phenomenon of *human care* (George 2002). She established the field of 'transcultural nursing' as a new field where professional nursing interacts with the concept of culture.

Since *Medical Communication Skills* aims at mobile doctors in a clinical setting, we have opted for the working term of *intercultural communication*, keeping in mind that the transcultural competence is the underlying model. To keep it simple, we use 'communicative competence' to refer to linguistic knowledge and skills as well as the underlying cultural knowledge and skills needed to function adequately and appropriately in a professional medical context.

1.2.3.5 Communication and Professional Status

If a language user has not acquired or learned the required pragmalinguistic resources—grammar, vocabulary, a repertoire of phrases and their appropriate use in the professional context—the end result may be misunderstanding, or even a communication breakdown (see, e.g. Basturkmen and Elder 2006 and Schnurr 2013). In a medical context, this can have negative consequences for others' perceptions of your professional status, because linguistic deficiencies can easily be interpreted as a lack of medical knowledge and skills or professional qualification. This can lead to conflicts and complaints, which may even threaten medical professionals' careers.

1.2.3.6 (Trans)cultural Organisational Management in Health Care

It is widely known and acknowledged that (trans)cultural organisational management is important. Concepts like 'diversity' include the idea that all people are different and that these differences can be used in a positive, productive way to ameliorate not only the working atmosphere and the well-being of **staff** in an organisation but that these differences can sometimes create competitive advantages.

Presently, there are several initiatives addressing standards in health care that seek to guarantee equality for all **patients** and to create more individualised options and offering for patients coming from different cultural backgrounds. The CLAS (National Standards for Culturally and Linguistically Appropriate Services in Health Care 2001) were created in the USA, but have also been recognised in Canada and Australia, and may be worth implementing as a way of promoting (trans)cultural competence in European health care. There is also the Amsterdam Declaration (EU) (2004): Hospitals of 12 European countries met in 2002 within the EU project *Migrant-Friendly Hospitals* to promote principles to improve transcultural health care and for a better treatment of international patients.

To show that culture is an intricate concept in medical communication, we would like to share the following finding from a Canadian study:

Sixty immigrant women with different cultural and ethnic backgrounds were asked what they most wanted doctors to understand about intercultural communication. The answer was that doctors should treat them first as *individuals* rather than as representatives of a cultural group.

As authors, we believe that treating people as individuals is the key to effective medical communication.

1.3   Communication and Mobility

1.3.1   Language-Discordant Doctor–Patient Communication

Language-discordant doctor–patient communication can either refer to the doctor or the patient speaking a different language. As both doctors and patients are increasingly mobile, more and more interactions are likely to be language-discordant. Ways of improving communication in language-discordant interactions include using professional health-care interpreters, medical mediators and/or bilingual doctors (Ferguson and Candib 2002; Pöchhacker and Shlesinger 2005) (see also Chap. 5).

1.3.2   Language-Discordant Doctor–Doctor Communication

Additionally, medical teams in the Western world increasingly consist of staff with diverse ethnic, cultural and linguistic backgrounds, as mobility among medical professionals increases (Jinks et al. 2000; Stilwell et al. 2004). This also increases the need for intercultural communication competence.

A study by Gasiorek and Van de Poel (2012) describes how mobile medical professionals working in European hospitals perceived their own communication with colleagues and how these colleagues perceived those professionals' communication in the host country's language. Its findings indicate a number of areas in which additional communication training would be useful, as well as important discrepancies between how the mobile medical professionals evaluated their communication, and how it is evaluated by their colleagues. Mobile medical professionals were generally confident in their communication skills and felt their colleagues saw them as confident. Colleagues, however, observed a number of communication problems—particularly related to cultural practices and nonverbal communication—of which mobile medical professionals appeared to be unaware. Given the growing number of mobile medical professionals in Western Europe and around the world, as well as the importance of effective medical communication to both patients and doctors, these issues demand attention.

1.3.3   Learning to Communicate

Communicative competence is something that can be taught and learned and can be adapted to any situation. They are not a fixed aspect of your personality; they are a knowledge and practice-based set of skills. There are a wealth of training courses (on paper and with professional trainers) that can help you improve your professional communication skills. However, the biggest challenge is to figure out how to incorporate these skills with your own personal preferences, communication style and personality.

   Medical Communication Skills is intended to increase your awareness of how doctor–patient communication works and how to make it more effective. It provides information and guidance about both the general consultation and a range of specific situations and cases and provides a range of example phrases, intercultural cases and approaches, so you can choose what suits your needs and your professional situation. The book thus functions as a medical performance support system and points at linguistic as well as cultural issues (see also, among others, Lu and Corbett 2012; Glendinning and Holmström 2002; Glendinning and Howard 2007; Parkinson 1999). Once you are aware of the basic framework and skills of these situations, observing yourself and colleagues will provide you with extra insights.

1.4   *Medical Communication Skills*: Five Chapters

In this first chapter, we have outlined the background of the book and introduced some terminology vital for understanding intercultural communication in a health-care context. In what follows, we will take a *patient-centred approach* to communication in health care (Chap. 2), in which both the doctor's and the patient's perspective on health will be centre of attention. In Chap. 3, we will focus on general communication skills that can be used across all the stages of the consultation, and then we narrow our focus to strategies used at specific points during the doctor–patient consultation (Chap. 4). The last chapter (Chap. 5) addresses challenging situations you may encounter with respect to the patient, content and communication channel. When and where appropriate, we will discuss intercultural challenges and suggest strategies to facilitate interaction with patients. At the end of every chapter, there are suggestions for additional reading on specific topics covered as well as a reference list. At the end of the book, we also provide a complete terminology list and an index.

You are welcome to read this book from cover to cover, but you can also pick a chapter or specific topics of interest from the table of contents or the index. You can also access a particular phrase or concept via the terminology list.

Additional Reading[1]

→ Cultural Challenges

Hall P, Keely E, Dojeiji S, Byszewski A, Marks M (2004) Communication skills, cultural challenges and individual support: challenges of international medical graduates in a Canadian healthcare environment. Medical Teacher 26:120–125

Jæger K (2012) Adopting a critical intercultural communication approach to understanding health professionals' encounter with ethnic minority patients. J Intercultural Commun August 2012:1404–1634

Schouten BC, Meeuwesen L (2006) Cultural differences in medical communication: a review of the literature. Patient Educ Couns 64 (1–3):21–34

→ Medical Communication as Language for Professional Purposes

Basturkmen H, Elder C (2006) The practice of LSP. In: Davies A, Elder C (eds) The handbook of applied linguistics. Blackwell Publishing, Oxford, pp 672–694

→ Medical Performance Support Systems

Glendinning EH, Holmström BAS (2002) English in medicine. A course in communication skills. Cambridge University Press, Cambridge

Glendinning EH, Howard R (2007) Professional English in use. Medicine. Cambridge University Press, Cambridge

Lu P, Corbett J (2012) English in medical education. An intercultural approach to teaching language and values. Multilingual Matters, Bristol

Parkinson J (1999) A manual of English for the overseas doctor. Churchill Livingstone, Edinburgh

→ Mobility

European Commission (2011) Mobility in Europe. http://ec.europa.eu/health-eu/care_for_me/mobility_in_europe

Jinks C, Ong BN, Paton C (2000) Mobile medics? The mobility of doctors in the European Economic Area. Health Policy 54:45–64

---

[1] The topics are given in alphabetical order.

OECD (2008) The looming crisis of the health workforce: How can OECD countries respond? [Datafile]. Retrieved from http://www.oecd.org/dataoecd/43/43/41522822.xls

Stilwell B, Diallo K, Zurn P, Vujicic M, Adams O, Dal Poz M (2004) Migration of healthcare workers from developing countries: strategic approaches to its management. Bull World Health Organ 82:595–600

References

Basturkmen H, Elder C (2006) The practice of LSP. In: Davies A, Elder C (eds) The handbook of applied linguistics. Blackwell Publishing, Oxford, pp 672–694

Berbyuk Lindström N (2008) Intercultural communication in health care. Non-Swedish physicians in Sweden. Gothenburg monographs in linguistics, vol 36. Department of Linguistics Dissertation, University of Gothenburg, Gothenburg

Bickley LS (2007) Bates' pocket guide to physical examination and history taking. Lippincott Williams & Wilkins, Philadelphia

Bickley LS, Szilagiy PG (2007) Bates' guide to physical examination and history taking. Lippincott Williams & Wilkins, Philadelphia

European Commission (2011) Mobility in Europe. http://ec.europa.eu/health-eu/care_for_me/mobility_in_europe

European Recommendations: The Amsterdam Declaration Towards Migrant Friendly Hospitals in an ethno-culturally diverse Europe (2004) http://www.mfh-eu.net/public/european_recommendations.htm. Accessed 20 Sept 2012

Ferguson WJ, Candib LM (2002) Culture, language, and doctor-patient relationship. Fam Med 34(5):353–361

Fiscella K, Frankel R (2000) Overcoming cultural barriers: international medical graduates in the United States. JAMA 283:1751

Fitzgerald H (2003) How different are we? Spoken discourse in intercultural communication. Multilingual Matters Ltd, Buffalo

Gasiorek J, Van de Poel K (2012) Divergent perspectives on language-discordant mobile medical professionals' communication with colleagues: an exploratory study. J Appl Commun Res 1–16. doi:10.1080/00909882.2012.712708

George JB (2002) Nursing theories: the base of professional nursing practice. Appleton and Lange, Norwalk

Gesensway D (2006) Handoff problems? Speak the same language as your colleagues. Today's Hospitalist. http://todayshospitalist.com/index.php?b_articles_read&cnt_168. Accessed July 2012

Glendinning EH, Holmström BAS (2002) English in medicine: a course in communication skills. Cambridge University Press, Cambridge

Glendinning EH, Howard R (2007) Professional English in use: medicine. Cambridge University Press, Cambridge

Hall P, Keely E, Dojeiji S, Byszewski A, Marks M (2004) Communication skills, cultural challenges and individual support: challenges of international medical graduates in a Canadian healthcare environment. Med Teach 26:120–125

Hewett DG, Watson BM, Gallois C, Ward M, Leggett BA (2009) Communication in medical records: intergroup language and patient care. J Lang Soc Psychol 28:119–138

Hornberger JC, Gibson CD, Wood W, Dequeldre C, Corso I, Palla B, Bloch DA (1996) Eliminating language barriers for non-English-speaking patients. Med Care 34(8):845–856

Hornberger K, Itakura H, Wilson SR (1997) Bridging language and cultural barriers between physicians and patients. Public Health Rep 112(5):410–417

Jinks C, Ong BN, Paton C (2000) Mobile medics? The mobility of doctors in the European Economic Area. Health Policy 54:45–64

Kurtz S, Silverman J, Draper J (2006) Teaching and learning communication skills in medicine. Radcliffe Publishing, Oxford

Lockyer J, Hofmeister M, Crutcher R, Klein D, Fidler H (2007) International medical graduates: learning for practice in Alberta, Canada. J Contin Educ Heal Prof 27:157–163

Lu P, Corbett J (2012) English in medical education: an intercultural approach to teaching language and values. Multilingual Matters, Bristol

McMahon GT (2004) Coming to America –international medical graduates in the United States. N Engl J Med 350:2435–2437

Moore RA, Rhodenbaugh EJ (2002) The unkindest cut of all: are international medical school graduates subjected to discrimination by general surgery residency programs? Curr Surg 59:228–236

National Standards for Culturally and Linguistically Appropriate Services in Health Care. Executive Summary (2001) U.S. Department of Health and Human Services, Office of Minority Health, Washington, DC

OECD (2008) The looming crisis of the health workforce: how can OECD countries respond? [Datafile]. Retrieved from http://www.oecd.org/dataoecd/43/43/41522822.xls

Parkinson J (1999) A manual of English for the overseas doctor. Churchill Livingstone, Edinburgh

Pendleton D, Schofield T, Tate P, Havelock P (2007) The new consultation: developing doctor-patient communication. Oxford University Press, Oxford

Pilotto LS, Duncan GF, Anderson-Wurf J (2007) Issues for clinicians training international medical graduates: a systematic review. Med J Aust 187:225–228

Pöchhacker F, Shlesinger M (2005) Discourse-based research on healthcare interpreting. Interpreting 7(2):157–165

Prabhu FR, Bickley LS (2007) Case studies to accompany Bates' guide to physical examination and history taking. Lippincott Williams & Wilkins, Philadelphia

Schnurr S (2013) Exploring professional communication: language in action. Routledge, Oxon/New York

Schouten BC, Meeuwesen L (2006) Cultural differences in medical communication: a review of the literature. Patient Educ Couns 64(1–3):21–34

Silverman J, Kurtz S, Draper J (2006) Skills for communicating with patients. Radcliffe Publishing, Oxford/San Francisco

Stewart MA (1995) Effective physician-patient communication and health outcomes: a review. Can Med Assoc J 15(9):1423–1433

Stilwell B, Diallo K, Zurn P, Vujicic M, Adams O, Dal Poz M (2004) Migration of healthcare workers from developing countries: strategic approaches to its management. Bull World Health Organ 82:595–600

Tate P (2007) The doctor's communication handbook. Radcliffe Publishing, Oxford

Travaline JM, Runchinskas R, D'Alonzo GE (2005) Patient-physical communication: why and how. J Am Osteopath Assoc Clin Pract 105(1):13–18

Watson BM, Hewett DG, Gallois C (2012) Intergroup communication and health care. In: Giles H (ed) The handbook of intergroup communication. Routledge, New York, pp 293–305

The Structure of the Consultation

2

Contents

K. Van de Poel et al., *Communication Skills for Foreign and Mobile Medical Professionals*,   13
DOI 10.1007/978-3-642-35112-9_2, © Springer-Verlag Berlin Heidelberg 2013

We will first describe the *patient-centred approach* to medicine. This approach results in a *dual track* consultation model, where doctors look at patients' problems from two perspectives: their own as well as the patient's.

In the *patient's agenda* or *perspective*

- ideas,
- concerns and
- expectations

play a central role.

After outlining these concepts, we will show how they are incorporated in the structure and *timeline of the consultation*.

Understanding and adopting this model of doctoring is of central importance for the mobile medical professional in today's Western world.

2.1   Concepts of Health

Already in 1946 the World Health Organisation defined being healthy not just as the absence of illness, health is a state of physical, mental and social well-being and not merely the absence of disease or infirmity. This definition forms the basis for different classifications used to define and measure the components of health. Following the WHO's 1986 *Ottawa Charter for Health Promotion,* health is a positive concept emphasising social and personal resources as well as physical capacities. Being healthy requires a balance of physical, mental and social well-being, sometimes referred to as the 'health triangle' (Nutter 2003).

Medical anthropology distinguishes between three health concepts indicating 'the absence of health':

- **Disease** is a pathological process, most often physical in nature. Examples of this are throat infections, cancer or schizophrenia. Although the origins of a disease are not always known, there is an element of objectivity about disease, because it is tangible: doctors are able to see, touch and measure it.
- **Illness** is the experience of feeling unhealthy. This is subjective and personal; it is a person's perception of their health, regardless of whether they in fact have a disease.
- **Sickness** is the external and public mode of not being healthy. Sickness is a social role, a state, a negotiated position in the world: it can be thought of as an 'agreement' between the person henceforward called 'sick' and a society which is prepared to recognise him as such.

These three concepts play a role when we define the interactants and their role in the consultation.

2.2   A Model of the Consultation

2.2.1   The Patient-Centred Model of Medicine

Medical care occurs in a context. Very simply put, the sequence of events leading up to a consultation is mainly patient-driven, since patients come to the consultation with certain beliefs and intuitions about what is wrong. They worry about what is going on and what is to come and have hopes and wishes for both the consultation and its outcomes. During the consultation, patient-related factors and doctor's understanding meet. They have an impact on and influence subsequent immediate, intermediate and long-term outcomes for both doctor and patient. This process has been termed the 'cycle of care' by Pendleton (1983).

Historically, in the consultation, doctors have practised what we would now call 'beneficent paternalism' (Tate 2007): when dealing with patients, doctors tended to act like well-meaning parents taking the lead in all of the consultation and making all the decisions. Although doctors have generally had their patients' best interests in mind, they had power over them in that they mainly focused on their own perspective and their own priorities. In the last 20–30 years, the patient has become more visible, and, consequently, medicine in the Western world has become increasingly *patient-oriented*. *Patient-oriented* or *patient-centred* medicine encourages doctors to consider both the doctor's and the patients' agenda (Mishler 1984; Campion et al. 1992; Epstein 2000). Closely related to this concept is the disease–illness model (Levenstein et al. 1989; Silverman et al. 2006; Stewart et al. 2003). This model proposes that there are two ways of talking about and understanding a condition: a disease framework, which takes a biomedical perspective, and an illness framework, which is guided by an individual's ideas, concerns and expectations (see Sect. 2.3.1). This gives rise to a *model* of consultation that seeks a balance between the doctor's and the patient's perspective, or between a disease-centred approach and an illness-centred approach. 'Balance' is the keyword here as Tate observes (2007, p. 10), 'The totally patient-centred doctor is probably a dangerous creature. Patients do after all come for medical advice and considered professional opinions. They do not expect the doctor to let them do all the talking, planning and managing.'

2.2.2   The Dual Track Model of Consultation

The dual track consultation model is also known as *the two-agendas model* or *two-perspectives model*. The key to this more patient-oriented approach is to follow not only your own biomedical agenda (as a doctor) but to also follow the patient's agenda. This means that you look at a patient's problem(s) not only from your own perspective as a medical professional but also from the patient's perspective. Thus, in short, you follow not only your own *doctor's track* but also the *patient's track*.

- **Doctor's track:** The doctor's information gathering agenda is based on traditional medical history taking, guided by the patient's complaint(s).
- **Patient's track:** No patient goes to a doctor with only a symptom. Before seeking a doctor's advice, patients always spend time thinking about their symptom(s).
  Generally, there are five types of questions in patient's mind. These cover the
  present (1), the past (2) and the future (3–5):
  1. Diagnosis:
     - *What is it?*
     - *What could be wrong?*
  2. Cause:
     - *What caused it?*
     - *Why has it happened?*
     - *Why did it happen to me?*
     - *Why now?*
  3. Prognosis:
     - *How long will it last?*
     - *Can it still get worse?*
  4. Effects:
     - *How has it affected me?*
     - *How will it affect me?*
  5. Treatment:
     - *Can it be cured?*
     - *If not, can it be controlled?*

These questions and their answers in the patient's mind are the real reasons that they
have come to see a doctor. They form the patient's agenda for the consultation and
reflect the patient's **illness** perspective, as opposed to the doctor's **disease** perspective (see Sect. 2.1 above). During history taking (the early phases of the consultation), there is a parallel search of these two frameworks by the doctor. In what
follows, we discuss how to address patients' needs alongside the doctor's typical
biomedical concerns.

2.3   The Patient's Frame of Reference

Concepts of health and illness have a strong **individual** component and rely on a
patient's own perspective and frame of reference (Sect. 2.3.1). Moreover, views on
health and illness differ considerably from **culture** to culture (Sect. 2.3.2). That is
one of the reasons why in the process of communication the views on what patients
and doctors may consider as 'being ill' may diverge (this will be discussed in greater
detail in Chap. 4).

   Our frame of reference is shaped by our upbringing, background and personal
experiences and includes our knowledge, experiences, opinions, values, norms,
needs, wishes and expectations. All of these determine our reality and how we
experience our interactions with others. We make our observations through this
frame and filter the messages others send us. This may only let through what

we already know, or what we like and want. We interpret and respond to what others say in terms of this frame of reference. Because frames of reference can differ, however, what is obvious or natural to you may not be obvious or natural to someone else, and this can result in misinterpretation and/or miscommunication.

Not being aware of your own frame of reference may first and foremost lead to drawing premature conclusions; not taking into account the other's frame of reference sufficiently may, among other things, make it more difficult to understand their wants and needs, and thus to interact with them positively and successfully.

2.3.1   The Patient's Health Perspective

As explained above, patients do not go to a doctor with just a symptom. Rather, they go to a doctor with **ideas** about their symptom(s), with **concerns** about their symptom(s) and with **expectations** related to their symptom(s). It is easier to understand and address the patient's perspective when you realise that they rely on these three dimensions also known as the *triad of ideas, concerns and expectations* or, in short, the *ICE* triad (as coined by Schofield, Havelock, Pendleton and Tate in 1979 (see Tate's personal evaluation of the concepts in 2007)):

- **Ideas (I)** are what patients think and feel about their health problem, its causes, its effects and its management. They are influenced by their ideas about health and health care (also called 'health understanding' or 'health beliefs') and about life and society in general (the patient's frame of reference; see Sect. 4.4.2).
- **Concerns (C)** are worries and fears about the problem, its implications and its effects on the patient's personal, family and occupational life.
- **Expectations (E)** are the information, the involvement and the care that they expect, hope or wish for and how they feel about these expectations.

Embedded in the ICE triad are the patient's **feelings** and emotions, as well as the **effects** of the problem **on their lives**. The combination of concerns and expectations has been shown to have a major influence on the patient's decision to consult a doctor.

2.3.2   The Cultural Component of Patient's Perspective

Even though many health-related concepts are well-defined (or feel that way to trained doctors), it is important to recognise that these concepts or beliefs may not be shared by everyone. Thus, it is also important to consider alternative health beliefs that patients may hold since they shape the consultation.

2.3.2.1   Social Beliefs

By way of example, we want to name three cultural components that shape the ICE triad: social beliefs, religious beliefs and attitudes. The following is taken from an intercultural study on health beliefs:

Social Beliefs
A study on health beliefs held by Ethiopians showed that a majority has faith
in traditional healers (Hodes 1997; see also Kleinman 1980). Other beliefs
included:
'… that epilepsy is caused by evil spirits, acquired by touching a seizing person and treated by smelling smoke from matches; that hepatitis is caused by a bat
or bird flying over a person and is treated with herbs; and that there are multiple
causes of diarrhoea, including journeying on a sunny day and jumping over diar-
rheal stool.' (Hodes 1997, p. 34)

It is quite easy to imagine how the communication between a Western doctor and
an Ethiopian patient could be difficult if the doctor is not aware of these beliefs.
Asking the patient to explain what it means for them to be healthy or ill can help
bridge some of the cultural differences and make patients feel that they are being
heard and cared for.

2.3.2.2 The Role of Religion in Health Behaviour

The religious background of the patient can influence his health behaviour in many
ways: if a patient believes, for example, that the will of God is manifesting itself in
their illness, they are likely to act differently than they would if they believe in the
idea of a self-determined life. Religious beliefs can also lead patients to reject certain kinds of treatments.

Religious background does have an impact not only on patients' concepts of
body, disease and sexuality but also on their daily routine, specific rituals (pictures
and statues of saints, praying, holidays), eating habits or a certain way of dealing
with pain, death and dying. It is important to keep in mind that patients may hold
specific views on medical measures influenced by their religion and the best way to
deal with them is with respect.

Specific strategies that can be adopted:

- Try to find out if your patients are religious, and if this affects their views on
  medical measures. Ask, for example, Is there a specific kind of religion important to you? If so, are there any rituals like praying or having special pictures or
  statues having near you in your room that would help you?
- Explore if there are any medical measures that would not be acceptable. Ask, for
  example, Is there any medical measure, such as a blood transfusion, that you
  wouldn't accept?
- If your patients express strong opinions about certain kinds of medical measures
  or treatment, ask them about the reasons behind their opinions. If you do not feel
  able to talk about certain religious thoughts with your patients, try to arrange for
  a person who will do so.

2.3.2.3 Attitudes About Preventive Health Care

People in different cultures may have different views on different aspects of medicine, **preventive medicine** being a case in point, and so patients from different cultural backgrounds may have different attitudes towards (and responses to) questions like:

- What is a healthy lifestyle?
- When and how do I seek medical care?
- Which preventive measures are good for me (and my children)?

The following is an illustration from an intercultural study:

Beliefs and Prevention

A study about knowledge and beliefs concerning preventive health care among Somali women in the USA (Carrol et al. 2007) found some similarities and some differences to Western women. Somali women shared many of beliefs of the Western world concerning preventive health care: The majority mentioned the importance of good sanitation, adequate nutrition, exercise and access to health care and medications for being healthy. On the other hand, most of the Somali women also talked about the role of traditional remedies, rituals and religion for staying healthy and recovering from illness (see Chap. 5). Many of the women surveyed also avoided use of tobacco and alcohol, not because they are seen as unhealthy but because these are expressly forbidden in the Koran.

Interestingly, almost none of them—despite having lived in the USA for a long time—were well informed about US preventive health services, such as Papanicolaou tests and mammography. Most women did not even recognise or understand the term 'cancer'.

Patients' attitudes to, for instance, prevention may also be determined by other factors. Cultures can differ in the degree to which they are oriented towards the present versus the future.[1] Patients in more **future-oriented** cultures (e.g. Asian cultures) are naturally more interested in preventive health care, such as regular check-ups, dental care, immunisations and screenings. Those in more **present-oriented** cultures (e.g. many African cultures), however, show less interest in preventative health care. The Somali women in the example above were more focused on their immediate survival than on their long-term or future health. They tended to describe their personal well-being as grounded in the present, here and now.

---

[1] This is a dimension of cultural difference observed by Hofstede (1997–2010). Although Hofstede's model of cultural differences has been subject to criticism, we believe its basic distinctions are helpful for understanding different perspectives on health issues.

2.4   Structuring the Consultation

Changes in society at large have given rise to a more balanced model of consultation that takes the patient's health perspective into account (as discussed above). We will now show how the two-perspectives model approach is incorporated in the structure and timeline of the consultation.

2.4.1   A Rationale for Structuring the Consultation

Structuring your consultation according to the outline that follows is beneficial to both you and your patients. However, to experience these benefits, you need to stick to this structure during the consultation. The key to doing this is to follow the structure in your mind throughout the consultation, using the outline below as a so-called mental map. A **consultation mental map** is a clear structure of the consultation to be kept in your mind at all times. Structuring the consultation using a mental map has the following **advantages**:

- It allows you to plan and think in terms of **outcomes** of the encounter, helping you stay focused on your goals.
- It allows you to make the organisation and progress of the consultation **overt** to you and your patient.
- For the **patient**, this overview facilitates their **involvement**, cooperation and satisfaction.
- Paradoxically, it enables **flexibility**: knowing what steps you have taken and what you still need to do provides you with confidence, which can help the consultation to flow freely.
- This flexibility can make you and your patient less uncertain, more **comfortable** and more relaxed. This helps make the consultation more pleasant and satisfactory for both parties.
- It also helps you to keep the **progress** of the consultation **under control**.
- It makes you more **attentive** to things that could derail the consultation and makes it easier for you to put the consultation back on the right track if needed. This 'safety net' can also allow you to look ahead with more confidence to difficult situations.
- It facilitates viewing communication problems as **challenges**, which you can learn to overcome with the right approach and techniques.
- It enables choosing the right communication **technique** at the right moment.
- And last but not least, it allows more efficient **time management**.

Beyond the consultation, following a clear structure:

- Facilitates reading and **taking notes**
- Facilitates **editing** reports and letters

There are a wide variety of verbal and nonverbal communication skills which indirectly contribute to structuring the consultation. Active listening, picking up and appropriately responding to cues, using a clear and understandable language, summarising and signposting, among others, all facilitate the structuring of the consultation. These skills are described in Chaps. 3 and 4.

2.4.2   Sequential Tasks

Structuring a consultation means **timing** and **sequencing** its different parts in a logi-cally ordered way. How each part is filled in depends mainly on the task(s) which has to be performed. Different conversations with different goals have different structures. Consultations in medicine occur in widely different contexts, from new to follow-up appointments; general practice clinics to hospital corridors; consulta-tion rooms to bedside communications; and short, simple encounters to long and complex ones. However, all consultations have some if not most major tasks in common.

Medical Communication Skills adopted the thesis that the clinician has five **sequential major tasks** to perform during a consultation (see the Calgary-Cambridge Guides initially developed by Kurtz and Silverman in 1996, and further developed by Kurtz, Silverman, Benson and Draper from 2003 onwards):

1. Initiating the session
2. Information gathering
3. The physical examination
4. Explaining and planning
5. Closing the session

Each of these major tasks involves a number of subtasks. Every subtask is, in turn, connected to specific communication skills. In the following chapters, we will sketch a communicative background for every subtask, highlight general and specific communication strategies and provide guidelines and tips where appropriate.

We follow the Calgary Cambridge Observation Guides and delineate and struc-ture the skills that have been shown by research and theory to aid doctor–patient communication. However, we have modified Silverman's structure of the consulta-tion slightly to allow information gathering to be as open and broad as possible from the very beginning of the consultation.

2.4.3   A Timeline of the Consultation

The first and last tasks in any consultation—greeting and saying goodbye—often take a set, formulaic format. Although greeting and saying farewell are formulaic interactions in every language, they are vital for establishing and maintaining rap-port with the patient. After these (formulaic) greetings, the middle section of the encounter forms the backbone of the consultation. This includes (1) information gathering, (2) physical examination and (3) explaining and planning the next steps. The final section of the consultation involves closing the session, which includes making plans to meet again as necessary, and saying farewell to the patient.

The following is an overview of the timeline of the consultation, with its five major sequential tasks:

1. Initiating the session
   Greeting the patient and establishing rapport

2. Information gathering
   Initiating information gathering
       Patients' narratives
       Exploring the patient's perspective and agenda
       Agenda screening
       Agenda setting
   Exploring the biomedical perspective
       Sequence of events
       Symptom analysis
       Relevant systems review
       Relevant background and context information
       General strategies for broaching sensitive topics
   Closing information gathering
3. The physical examination
4. Explaining and planning
   Explaining the (differential) diagnosis–hypothesis
   Explaining the management plan
       Negotiating to arrive at a mutually accepted management plan
       Enabling the patient to implement the management plan
5. Closing the session
   Forward planning
   Providing a point of closure
   Saying goodbye

2.5   Summary

In the next three chapters, we will discuss the communication skills needed to make the consultation as smooth and positive as possible. Chapter 3 will focus on general strategies and communication skills used throughout the consultation. Chapter 4 will take the sequential tasks as a starting point for a discussion of the verbal and nonverbal communication skills used in each task. Finally, Chap. 5 will review and discuss strategies for addressing challenges specific to this medical context.

Additional Reading

→ The Disease-Illness Model

Gwyn R (2002) Communicating health and illness. Sage Publications, London/Thousand Oaks/ New Delhi

Levenstein JH, Belle Brown J, Weston WW, Stewart M, McCracken EC, McWhinney I (1989) Patient-centred clinical interviewing. In Stewart M, Roter D (eds.) Communicating with medical patients. Sage Publications, Inc., Newbury Park

Stewart M, Belle Browne J, Wayne Weston W, McWhinney IR, McWilliam CL, Freeman TR (2003) Patient-centred medicine: transforming the clinical method. Sage, Thousand Oaks

→ Health Literacy

Elder C, Barber M, Staples M, Osborne RH, Clerehan R, Buchbinder R (2012) Assessing health literacy: a new domain for collaboration between language testers and health professionals. Language Assessment Quarterly: An International Journal 9(3):205–224

→ Intercultural Health Beliefs

Hodes RM (1997) Cross-cultural medicine and diverse health beliefs. Ethiopians abroad. West J Med 166:29–36
Sorajjakool S, Carr MF, Nam J (2009) World Religions for healthcare professionals. Routledge, New York

→ The Patient-Centred Model of Medicine

Campion PD, Butler NM, Cox AD (1992) Principal agendas of doctors and patients in general practice consultations. J Fam Pract 9:181–190
Epstein RM (2000) The science of patient-centred care. J Fam Pract 49:805–807
Mishler EG (1984) The discourse of medicine: dialectics of medical interviews. Ablex, Norwood
Pendleton D, Schofield T, Tate P, Havelock P (2007) The new consultation. Developing doctor–patient communication. Oxford University Press, Oxford

→ Preventive Health Care

Betancourt JR, Carillo JE, Green AR, Maina A (2004) Barriers to health promotion and disease prevention in the Latino population. Clinical Cornerstone 6:16–26
Carrol J, Epstein R, Fiscella K, Volpe E, Diaz K, Omar S (2007) Knowledge and beliefs about health promotion and preventive health care among Somali women in the United States. Health Care Women Int 28(4):360–380
Naish J, Brown J, Denton B (1994) Intercultural consultations: investigation of factors that deter non-English speaking women from attending their general practitioners for cervical screening. Br Med J 309:1126–1128

→ Skills for Communicating with Patients

Kurtz SM, Silverman JD, Draper J (2006) Teaching and learning communication skills in medicine. Radcliffe Medical Press, Oxford
Kurtz S, Silverman J, Benson J, Draper J (2003) Marrying content and process in clinical method teaching: enhancing the Calgary-Cambridge guides. Acad Med 78(8):802–809
Silverman JD, Kurtz SM, Draper J (2006) Skills for communicating with patients. Radcliffe Publishing, Oxford/San Francisco

→ The Triad of Ideas, Concerns and Expectations

Nutter S (2003) The health triangle. Anchor Points, Inc., s.l.
Pendleton D (1983) Doctor-patient communication: a review. In Pendleton D and Hasler J (eds) Doctor-patient communication. Academic Press, London
World Health Organization. The Ottawa Charter for Health Promotion. Adopted at the First International Conference on Health Promotion, Ottawa, 21 November 1986—WHO/HPR/HEP/95.1.

References

Campion PD, Butler NM, Cox AD (1992) Principal agendas of doctors and patients in general practice consultations. J Fam Pract 9:181–190
Carrol J, Epstein R, Fiscella K, Volpe E, Diaz K, Omar S (2007) Knowledge and beliefs about health promotion and preventive health care among Somali women in the United States. Health Care Women Int 28(4):360–380
Epstein RM (2000) The science of patient-centred care. J Fam Pract 49:805–807
Hodes RM (1997) Cross-cultural medicine and diverse health beliefs. Ethiopians Abroad. West J Med 166:29–36
Kleinman A (1980) Patients and healers in the context of culture. University of California Press, Berkeley
Kurtz SM, Silverman JD (1996) The Calgary-Cambridge Referenced Observation Guides: an aid to defining the curriculum and organizing the teaching in communication training programmes. Med Educ 30(2):83–89
Kurtz SM, Silverman JD, Draper J (1998) Teaching and learning communication skills in medicine. Radcliffe Medical Press, Oxford
Kurtz S, Silverman J, Benson J, Draper J (2003) Marrying content and process in clinical method teaching: enhancing the Calgary-Cambridge Guides. Acad Med 78(8):802–809
Levenstein JH, Belle Brown J, Weston WW, Stewart M, McCracken EC, McWhinney I (1989) Patient-centred clinical interviewing. In: Stewart M, Roter D (eds) Communicating with medical patients. Sage Publications Inc, Newbury Park
Mishler EG (1984) The discourse of medicine: dialectics of medical interviews. Ablex, Norwood
Nutter S (2003) The health triangle. Anchor Points, Inc., s.l.
Pendleton D (1983) Doctor-patient communication: a review. In: Pendleton D, Hasler J (eds) Doctor-patient communication. Academic, London
Silverman JD, Kurtz SM, Draper J (2006) Skills for communicating with patients. Radcliffe Publishing, Oxford/San Francisco
Stewart M, Belle Browne J, Wayne Weston W, McWhinney IR, McWilliam CL, Freeman TR (2003) Patient-centred medicine: transforming the clinical method. Sage, Thousand Oaks
Tate P (2007) The doctor's communication handbook. Radcliffe Publishing, Oxford
World Health Organization (1986) The Ottawa charter for health promotion. Adopted at the first international conference on health promotion, WHO/HPR/HEP/95.1, Ottawa, 21 Nov 1986

General Communication Strategies and Skills

3

Contents

What to Expect in This Chapter
In communication, little things can make a big difference. This chapter focuses on general communication skills that you can use across all stages of a patient consultation. Specifically, we discuss:
- Attentive and active listening
- Appropriate verbal and nonverbal language use
- Building rapport
We will first consider how listening underlies all communication. Then we will discuss the interplay between the different modes of communication. Finally, we will consider how communication can strengthen the professional relationships that you engage in.
All of these skills will help you be a better and more effective communicator in your clinical work.

3.1   Active Listening

3.1.1   Active or Attentive Listening

Good listening is active listening. Active listening is the first step to effective communication and involves being attentive and responsive:
- **Being attentive** means paying attention to what the speaker is saying and doing, both verbally and nonverbally.
- **Being responsive** means reacting appropriately to the verbal and nonverbal messages you receive, showing your listener that you are paying attention to and understanding them.

3.1.2   The Skills Used in Active Listening

Active listening involves a number of different, specific skills that help **facilitate**, **direct** and **structure** your interaction with others (Fassaert et al. 2007; Wiseman 1995; Witte and Morrison 1995). Using these skills makes communication more effective and more satisfying for both you and your patients. Below, we discuss them in terms of their primary function (facilitating, directing or structuring), though any of these skills may be used during any part of the consultation.

3.1.2.1 Facilitative Skills
Facilitative skills include (non)verbal encouragement, silence, repetition, paraphrasing, reflecting feelings, picking up and responding to cues.
- **Nonverbal Encouragement**
  We show others that we are paying attention to them mainly through the feedback we give them. Showing that we are paying attention communicates interest and respect and reassures speakers that we care about them as people. Often, the

feedback we use to indicate that we are paying attention is nonverbal: rather than saying, 'I'm listening', we show others that we are doing so through actions like eye contact and body posture (Beattie 2003):

– **Eye Contact**

In most Western cultures, making eye contact demonstrates that you are listening and provides encouragement for the other person to keep speaking. Regular eye contact also tells them that you sympathise with their situation and that you feel comfortable with them.

Eye contact does not necessarily mean looking continuously into a person's eyes, or staring at them. Doing this may make a speaker feel uncomfortable. Often, positioning yourself at angle can help create a situation where you can focus your attention on the speaker without making them uncomfortable.

In addition to facilitating conversation, eye contact can also help direct the flow of conversation. A meaningful look can communicate that one person wants to say something, or that it is time for them to stop and let the other speaker to take over again.

– **Body Posture and Movements**

Relaxed body posture can also communicate attention and encourage a speaker to continue. Encouraging and relaxed posture includes leaning forward slightly, nodding regularly and/or discretely gesturing for the patient to keep speaking. It is important that such movements be subtle enough not to distract the patient. It is best to avoid fiddling, squirming or tapping your fingers, as well as other related movements. Patients may interpret this as a signal of boredom or a lack of attention.

• **Verbal Encouragement**

We also show others we are paying attention through our use of verbal encouragement. Examples of this include expressions like, 'I see', 'uh huh' and 'go on'. These phrases are usually short and neutral. Their function is to acknowledge patients, their story and their feelings and let patients know that you are listening, without interrupting the flow of their speech.

• **Use of Silence**

Sometimes, silence can be used to facilitate conversation. Silences usually have a reason:

– A patient may first want time to think, to reorder their ideas or to figure out how to express their thoughts.

– A patient may have been touched emotionally, or offended, by something that has been said (e.g. if a topic is linked to a social taboo).

– A patient may feel that they have nothing more to say about a particular topic.

Often, you can guess the patient's reason for silence using clues from the context. Here, short verbal questions may also help you determine the reason for the silence. Different responses are appropriate for different reasons for silence:

– For patients that are trying to organise their thoughts, a short question inviting them to continue, such as 'Can you tell me more about this?' or 'What are you thinking about this', can be helpful.

- For patients that are working through emotions associated with what was been said, it can be helpful to provide a sympathetic comment such as 'I have the impression that you find it difficult to tell more about this', with a friendly, understanding and inviting tone.
- For patients who have nothing more to say, the best answer can be to change the subject of discussion.
- If you are not sure of the reason for silence, it can be best to ask an open question such as 'May I ask you, as this may be difficult: what makes it difficult for you?' or 'Is there anything else you would like to tell me?'

If you need to be silent for a period of time, let the patient know. You can make a comment explaining the silence, such as 'I just want to think over all you have been telling' or 'I first want to make some notes'.

There can be a fine line between comfortable and uncomfortable silence. To make sure everyone has time to process and think about what is being said, a good general rule is to wait at least 3–5 s before intervening or responding if there is a pause in conversation.

- **Repetition (Echoing)**

Repeating or echoing (one of) the last few words of patients' sentences when they pause can **encourage** them to keep talking. Echoing the patient's own words not only shows that you are listening and understanding them but also enables them to hear what they have just said. This can help them refocus and make sure they are communicating what they intend:

The patient says:	You echo:
– ... *Then I suddenly felt something strange in my stomach ...*	– *In your stomach?*

This strategy should be used in moderation. Frequent echoing may be irritating, as patients may think you are parroting or mocking them. One way to avoid the impression that you are parroting is to repeat the key ideas or essence of what you heard in your own words. (This is referred to as *paraphrasing*; see below.)

Repetition can also be a useful technique to reinforce information when explaining a diagnosis to a patient and planning next steps in treatment or management. In this case, you may repeat your own words to emphasise important points or may echo the patient's words to confirm understanding.

- **Paraphrasing**

Paraphrasing means restating what you have heard and understood in your own words. Paraphrasing can be a good way to check whether your own interpretation of what a patient has said is accurate. By playing back the message in your own words, you show the patient what you have understood. Following your paraphrasing with a short phrase like 'Is this correct?' gives the patient the opportunity to correct any misunderstandings and to embellish the story further if they would like to.

The process of paraphrasing involves eliciting, organising and reflecting on the information a patient provides. This process is something both you and your patients can learn from.

- **Reflecting Feelings**
  While paraphrasing generally refers to the content of what the other was saying, reflecting feelings involves summarising and playing back your impression of the feelings or emotions that others are experiencing. This is often done through short questions or phrases such as 'It seems that you're upset by this'. As with paraphrasing content, you may follow such a statement with a short question like 'Is that correct?' to check that you have understood the patient properly. Reflecting feelings can also help you empathise with patients and see the situation from their perspective.

- **Picking Up and Responding to Cues**
  Cues are **signals** by one person that are picked up by another. During a medical consultation, they generally point to patient's emotions, ideas, concerns and expectations.
  Cues can be both verbal and nonverbal:

Examples of **verbal cues**:	**Nonverbal cues** can be found in the patient's:
– *I feel worse.* (incomplete message)	– *Tone of voice* (signalling, e.g. distress)
– *It doesn't improve.* (vague message)	– *Facial expression* (signalling, e.g. depression)
– *I have problems.* (emotional message)	– *Eye movement* (signalling, e.g. boredom)
– *It is always like that.* (generalisation)	– *Posture* (signalling, e.g. dislike)

Picking up verbal and nonverbal cues requires **care and attention**. A doctor cannot ignore patients' cues: these cues are requests for help or for a response. Rather, a doctor must decide whether to act on the cue immediately or wait and respond later. Regardless of whether the issue which a cue signal can be addressed immediately, it is important to acknowledge the cue, either verbally or nonverbally.

Examples of **verbal cues**:	Acknowledgement:
I feel worse.	→ *Worse than what? In what sense? About what? …*
It doesn't improve.	→ *What doesn't improve? …*
I have problems.	→ *Do you care to tell me about them? …*
It is always like that.	→ *Does that mean every month? …*

Acknowledging a cue shows the patient that you have seen or heard what they are trying to communicate, and in doing so acknowledges patients' right to have their own views and feelings, even if you disagree. This can facilitate present and future communication, as well as help build rapport (see Sect. 3.4).

Reflecting feelings is one way of acknowledging and responding to cues. As mentioned above, it can also help you empathise with your patient and see the situation from that patient's perspective:

Instead of …	Say …
– *Yes but …* (a response which is easily perceived as a negation of the acceptance and may provoke defensiveness)	→ *Yes, I understand …* (an accepting response followed by an attentive silence inviting the patient to continue)

3.1.2.2 Directive Skills

Directive skills are powerful tools in medical interaction. They include asking questions, asking for clarifications, providing a rationale and signposting.

- **Asking Questions**
  Asking good questions provides evidence that you are a good listener. As with all types of communication, it is important to consider both **content** (what you say) and **language** (how you say it) when formulating a question.

The **content** of a good question:

- **Fits in the conversation** and relates directly to the patient's story. A good question should not be unexpected or unrelated to what has come before. If you need to change topics, let your patient know by signposting (see Sect. 3.1.2.2 on p. 33).

- **Follows the *open-to-closed cone of questioning*:** A good general strategy for gathering information from patients is to start with open-ended questions and move towards more focused and closed-ended questions.

  - *Open questions* are very broad, giving the patient a lot of freedom to choose how they respond. It is important to use open questions when exploring a new problem. Open questions allow patients to provide much more information than closed questions. They also give patients the opportunity to reflect and think and to tell a story (or narrative) about the problem they are experiencing:

  - *Tell me …*.
  - *Tell me about …*
  - *What happened? …*
  - *What do you think about …?*
  - *How did …?*
  - *What are your intentions to …?*

– **Focused or directed questions**, which generally follow open questions, allow you to ask for clarification or additional information about points that have been brought up in response to open questions:

> – *Does something make your headaches change, for better or worse?*

– **Closed questions** are very focused questions and are used to get specific pieces of information you consider important. These are generally asked last and used to clarify or understand details of patients' problems:

> – *Is it a sharp pain?*

The **language** of a good question:
* **Is language that a patient can understand** (see *Appropriate verbal communication—Understandable language* Sect. 3.2.1). This generally means using understandable, respectful and clear language and avoiding medical jargon.
* **Is structured** in a way that makes it clear how to provide an answer:

Instead of …	Say …
– *Do you feel better or do you still feel the pain?* (a double question)	→ *Do you feel better now?* (a single question)
– *Do you feel the pain? When do you feel the pain? How long does it last?* (many sequential closed questions)	→ *Sorry, to be complete, I now have to ask a series of short questions. A 'yes' or 'no' is OK.* (announce the questions, explain why and apologise)
– *Is the pain sharp or dull or throbbing?* (multiple choice question excluding other answers)	→ *Please tell me more about the pain. What kind of pain is it?* or: *Was it a sharp pain?* (simple questions)

* **Uses descriptive and non-judgmental language** (see *Appropriate Verbal Communication—Respectful Language* Sect. 3.2.2)). This generally means using words and terms that describe the problem at hand in a neutral way rather than in a way that suggests an opinion or evaluation of a given behaviour:

Instead of …	Say …
Suggestive questions:	More tactful questions:
– *You probably also suffer from …?* (inherent judgment and disapproval)	→ *What you just mentioned may cause other problems … Are you experiencing any other problems?* (descriptive, non–judgmental question)
– *Can't you try …?* (inherent judgment and disapproval)	→ *One option could be to try to …* (non–judgmental advice)
– *Why didn't you go on taking the new drug?* (a why question which easily sounds disapproving, accusing or condemning)	→ *Can you tell me about your experience with the new drug?* (descriptive, non–judgmental question)
– *Do you drink a lot?* (overtly direct or confrontational question)	→ *How would you describe your use of alcohol?* (a descriptive, non–judgmental question)

- **Asking for Clarification**
  Although you often ask questions to gain new information, sometimes questions are needed to **clarify information** that a patient has already provided. This is usually necessary when a patient's statements are too vague or require further elaboration before you can use the information they are trying to provide:

The patient says …	You respond …
– *I feel bad.*	→ *What feels bad?*
– *This uncertainty is driving me crazy.*	→ *What makes you feel uncertain?*

Echoing or paraphrasing (see above p. 28) what was unclear, or reflecting feelings, may precede the clarifying questions as an introduction:

- *You said that … Could you give an example?*
- *That must have been difficult for you. Could you tell me more about it?*

Asking questions related to time frame may be useful to clarify the sequence of events, when this is important:

The patient says …	You respond …
– *Since I left hospital ….*	→ *When exactly did you leave the hospital?*

- **Providing a Rationale (Sharing Thoughts)**
  Providing a rationale means sharing your **reasons** for your actions and questions with the patient. Explaining why you want to know things is a sign of respect to the patient and helps them understand why you are doing what you do or asking what ask. Providing a rationale is also an excellent way to encourage them to provide you with better, more complete information and to help patients feel involved in the process of the consultation:

  – *Earlier on you mentioned nausea. I now would like to know more about it. When did it start?*

- **Signposting**
  A 'signpost' is an explicit **statement** telling someone what you are about to say or do. Signposts are often used to transition or change directions during a conversation or consultation. They draw attention to your verbal and nonverbal behaviour and make clear to the patient what is going to happen next. Making clear what is going to happen next can help reduce some of the uncertainty and anxiety a patient may be feeling, give patients a greater sense of control and help put them at ease.

  A signpost may include the rationale (see above) for the next step or subject in a consultation:

  – *In order to understand this, I first want to know if it is related to your meals. Can you tell me if …?*
  – *I would now like to know more about …*

Signposting can also help you structure the consultation and your interactions more generally. This is a form of meta-communication (see Sect. 3.1.2.3 p. 35 below).

3.1.2.3 Structuring Skills

Finally, structuring skills include chunking and checking, timing the information, explicitly highlighting particular information, summarising, structuring and using meta-communication.

- **Chunking and Checking**

  'Chunking' means breaking down longer and more complex explanations into **digestible pieces,** or 'chunks'. This can help both patient understanding and recall, because smaller pieces of information are easier to process.

  After you give each piece of information, check that patients have understood before moving on to the next piece of information. You may do this by asking explicitly or by observing patients' nonverbal responses. Only move on to the next 'chunk' when you are confident a patient has understood the previous chunk:

  - *I will now tell you what I **think is wrong**,*
    *then what I **expect to happen** and*
    *finally what **can be done.***

- **Timing Information**

  Sometimes, *when* you provide a piece of information can be as important as *what* you say. Research shows that we are better at remembering what we are told first (the primacy effect) and what we have been told last (the recency effect), than what has come in between. So, if you have something important to tell a patient, consider saying it either at the beginning or at the end of your discussion with them.

- **Explicit Highlighting**

  Explicit highlighting means verbally **drawing attention** to a particular point. This can be similar to signposting but makes explicit that what follows is something that requires attention. This is a form of meta-communication (see p. 35 below):

  - *The most important thing is …*
  - *I am going to tell you what I think is wrong …*

- **Summarising**

  Summarising is closely related to **paraphrasing**, but it is often more extensive. Summarising generally restates all of the important points in a discussion up to that point rather than just reformulating the most recent statement:

  - *Can I just see if this is right? You first … is that right?*

  Sometimes, it can be helpful to signpost a summary:

  - *Let's see whether we've discussed everything. First, …*
  - *Now that we have summarised our talk so far, we can …*

Like paraphrasing, summarising may be used to check your understanding of what the patient has said. It can also give patients an explicit opportunity to elaborate on or extend their story. This can enhance accuracy and help patients provide the most complete information possible. Asking short questions such as 'Is that correct?' or 'Would you still like to add something?' can facilitate this. Be aware that although summarising is helpful, doing it too frequently can disrupt the flow of communication.

- **Structuring**
Structuring means **sequencing** actions in an ordered way. Having a plan for the structure of an interaction can help make your conversations smoother and can help you make sure you have not missed anything important.

For medical consultations, it can be helpful to have a mental map—that is, a plan of how something will go—not only for the entire consultation but also for different subparts of this process. Mental maps help provide a clear structure of the content to be kept in mind during each part of the interaction. The basic outline of the consultation (with its five tasks) presented in Chap. 2 is one example of a mental map.

- **Meta-communication**
Meta-communication literally means **communication about** communication. In doctor–patient communication, it usually refers to communication about how the consultation is going to proceed and what is going to be discussed or done next. Both signposting and explicit highlighting (discussed above) are forms of meta-communication.

Meta-communication may be verbal or nonverbal. You can explicitly state what you will do or talk about next (as in signposting), or you may communicate these intentions with nonverbal signals like eye contact, facial expression or tone of voice (see Sects. 3.3.3.3, 3.3.2.1 and 3.3.3.4).

In cases where communication has stalled or otherwise become difficult, you can use meta-communication to try to understand how the problem has come about and how best to solve it or proceed in a new direction. Thus, meta-communication can also be used to prevent or solve *conflicts* with patients in the consultation (Makoni 1998), as discussed in Chap. 5 (Sect. 3.5).

3.2 Appropriate Verbal Communication

How we say things can be as important as *what* we say. The same basic message can be interpreted very differently if it is said in different ways. Using appropriate language helps both you and the patient have an effective and satisfying consultation (see Pendleton et al. 2007; Silverman et al. 2006; Tate 2007). Generally, appropriate language is **understandable** (Sect. 3.2.1), **respectful** (Sect. 3.2.2) and **honest** (Sect. 3.2.3).

3.2.1 Understandable Language

Understandable language uses simple, recognisable and clear words and phrases to ask questions, explain and plan.

- **Simple** language avoids jargon, abbreviations and other difficult or complex words and phrases:

Instead of …	Say …
– *Do you feel better or do you still feel the pain?* (a double question)	→ *Do you feel better? (single question)*
– *Is the pain sharp or dull or throbbing?* (too many sequential closed questions or multiple choice questions)	→ *Is it a sharp pain? (single question)*

Sometimes such language cannot be avoided. In this case, it is best to apologise for the complex language and then do what you can to help make this complex language easier for the patient to understand. Some strategies for doing this are:
- Breaking long explanations down into smaller, more digestible 'chunks' (see above Sect. 3.1.2.3). Check that the patient has understood each chunk before moving on to the next:

> – *I will tell you what I think is wrong, then what I expect to happen and finally what can be done.*

- Using logical structuring to make these chunks easier to understand and to connect to each other:

> – *I will **first** tell you what I think is wrong, **then** what I expect to happen and **finally** what can be done.*

- Using explicit categorisation to make these chunks easier to understand and to connect to each other:

> – *I will now tell you what **I think is wrong**, then what I **expect to happen** and finally what **can be done**.*

- **Recognisable** language uses words and phrases that the patient knows. This can mean adapting your language to the individual patient. This may include:
  - Using the same words or expressions you hear the patient using. This helps show them that you are listening and understand what they are saying to you:

A child says …	You say …
– I felt a pain in my tummy …	*→ In your tummy? …*

- Trying to match the rate of speed of a patient's speech.
- Using language at the same level of complexity they are using:

Instead of replying to the question …	Say …
– What about my knee, doctor?	*→ I think you have some wear*
– I think you have early arthritis.	*and tear, with a little early*
	arthritis.

- **Clear** language uses concrete words and phrases, rather than ambiguous ones:
  - **Vague** words to be avoided are:

  > *– a little bit, common, possible, rare, …*
  > *– conditional expressions like: as is usual, in theory*

  - **Ambiguities** to be avoided are:
    Percentages or other figures, which patients may interpret in a different way. Such information is best conveyed in ways that are meaningful to the individual patient without manipulating the message. A risk reduction may be statistically significant, but individually insignificant (or vice versa).
    Words and phrases like *don't worry* that may mean something different to the patient than they do to you.
    Misleading phrases like *a tiny injection* to make something sound less threatening, but may set expectations unfairly:

Instead of …	Say …
– Don't worry.	*→ It is only a minor infection. I will*
	prescribe you some medication.

  - To the extent possible, clear language also provides **explanations** or **rationales** for why what you say is true or important:

Instead of …	Say …
– *Everyone knows that this is wrong. (generalisation)*	→ *There is evidence that following a heart attack, giving up smoking may double longevity. (correct facts and views)*
– *You know that I am opposed to smoking. (authoritative or dogmatic reasoning—proof by intimidation)*	
– *Smoking is bad. Of course you should have given up smoking a long time ago because it is unhealthy. (circular reasoning)*	→ *Cutting out fatty foods may improve your cholesterol. (relevant arguments)*

– Different cultures may have different **communication styles**.
Some cultures use metaphorical language to express their feelings, wishes, ideas and experiences (Ruthrof 2000; Yu 2009). For example, in Arabic, it is common to express requests like 'I would like to rest a little bit' using elaborate, metaphorical language.

In some cultures, people may use particular illustrations, images or comparisons to describe their feelings. In Arabic, for example, one might say 'Doctor, I cannot distinguish my head from the garden fence', an expression which simply means that a patient feels confused.

In your own speech, try to avoid metaphors, figures of speech and proverbs to avoid confusion. Use clear language.

Body parts are often used to describe feelings and states of mind. However, many of these expressions do not translate directly, so it is important to take care when using them. Some examples:

Metaphor	Meaning
– English: *He is wearing his **heart** on his sleeve.*	→ *He doesn't think a lot before talking. He speaks easily about what he is thinking.*
– German: *Sie nimmt ihn auf den **Arm**.*	→ Literal translation: *She is taking him on his arm.* Meaning: *She is pulling his **leg**. She is teasing him.*
– French: *Il lui casse les **reins**.*	→ Literal translation: *He is breaking his kidneys.* Meaning: *He is breaking his **back**. He is destroying his strength of character.*

3.2.2 Respectful Language

Respectful language makes communication more effective in many ways. It is one of the best ways to prevent misunderstandings and conflicts. It also reassures patients that you see them as *people* who have personal and social needs as well as medical needs. Respectful language shows attention, uses descriptive words and is problem-oriented.

- **Showing attention** demonstrates that you are interested and engaged in what is being said, which is also a sign of respect. Showing attention is also an important part of *active listening*, discussed above.
- **Using descriptive words**, rather than judgmental words, allows you to ask questions and gather information in a way that makes a patient feel respected and comfortable, rather than judged:

Instead of ...	Say ...
– *What about my knee, doctor?*	→ *I think you have some wear and*
– *You're overweight and that's why you have knee pain. (not respectful)*	*tear, with a little early arthritis.*
– *This is wrong. (accusation)*	→ *This may have negative consequences.*
– *You're probably also suffering from ... (suggestive question containing an inherent assumption of judgment and disapproval)*	→ *What you just mentioned may cause suffering... If this is the case, can you tell me how it makes you feel?*

- Here, choice of words and phrases is very important: it is best to choose words that say or ask what something is without suggesting an opinion or evaluation (either positive or negative) of it, or suggesting particular intentions on the part of the patient:

Instead of ...	Say ...
calling a child *attention–seeking*	→ *The child is attention–liking.*

- *Why questions* may make patients think you are suspicious of them or their reasons for doing things. Patients might experience these questions as accusatory or disapproving. This could make patients feel as if they have to 'defend' themselves, and could lead them to feel uncomfortable and/or to invent reasons for their actions:

Instead of …	Say …
– *Why didn't you go on taking the new drug?*	→ *Can you tell me about your experience with the new drug? (more tactful using a descriptive non–judgmental language)*

- Overtly direct or confrontational questions may also make patients think you disapprove of their behaviour:

Instead of …	Say …
– *Do you drink a lot?*	→ *How would you describe your use of alcohol? (more respectful using a descriptive non–judgmental language)*

- Pseudo-questions and presuppositions may also make patients think you are judging them, and are best replaced with more descriptive statements:

Instead of …	Say …
– *Do you ever think you'll come off the tranquillisers?*	→ *Changing habits is difficult for everybody. We should have a plan … (more tactful using a descriptive non–judgmental language)*

- **Problem-oriented** language focuses on the patient's medical issue, in a way that is clear and understandable to them. Here, a stepwise approach is often helpful. A stepwise approach involves approaching a problem in steps or phases and providing *provisional or optional statements* with a *rationale*:

Instead of …	Say …
– *Your blood pressure is up. I will prescribe you some tablets. Take one a day. (controlling)*	→ *I think your blood pressure needs treatment. Here is a leaflet on the topic. I would like you to come back to discuss the treatment once you have had the chance to look it over. (more tactful using a problem–oriented stepwise approach)*

Problem-oriented language also uses words and phrases that a patient can understand (see *understandable language*, Sect. 3.2.1 above), and by involving the patient in decisions about treatment and care.

3.2.3   Honest Language

Honest language is above all things truthful. Doctors always have to be honest with their patients, even when this is difficult. This includes being truthful about the seriousness of their diagnosis, their options for treatment and their prognosis. This is closely related to both understandable and respectful language. Generally, honest language is also clear (not vague or ambiguous) and descriptive (non-judgmental).

Different cultures may have different perspectives towards honesty in medical settings.

In some cultures, it may be considered appropriate to comfort patients by telling them positive things, even if they are not (completely) true. In this case, supporting patients psychologically is considered to be a higher priority than telling them the truth.

In most Western countries, it is considered important to be completely honest with the patients about their state and prognosis. In these cultures, it is not considered appropriate to say 'I am sure it's going to be fine' to a patient who is terminally ill. Being honest to patients without intimidating or depressing them can be very challenging.

- **Strategies**
  - Try to find out in each case what kind of emotional support your patients need and want by observing them carefully and listening attentively. It is possible to be both honest and emotionally supportive.
  - Ask your patients, What can I do for you now? How can I help you? Is there anyone you would like to call? Their answers can tell you whether they are seeking (honest) information, or emotional support.

3.3   Appropriate Nonverbal Communication

How we say things can be as important as *what* we say. While the focus of our verbal communication (discussed in the previous section) is generally the content of our messages, our **attitudes** about what we say are often communicated through our nonverbal communication (see, for instance, Beattie 2003; Fernández 2010; Watzlawick et al. 2011). Nonverbal information helps us understand the meaning of what others say: the same words said in a different tone of voice (e.g. angry compared to cheerful) can have a very different meaning. Thus, it is important to be aware of your nonverbal communication when communicating with patients.

3.3.1   Consistency

In most cases, our nonverbal behaviour supports our verbal behaviour. In other words, we try to send the same message through both verbal and nonverbal channels.

However, if the two contradict each other—with words saying one thing, while non-verbal behaviour suggests another—people tend to believe the *nonverbal* message more than the verbal message. To the extent possible, it is best to avoid such contradictory communication, as it may cause confusion. Such communication may also undermine others' trust and belief in our sincerity and honesty. Think about how differently you would understand the following message depending on how it is said, for example:

What is said …	How it is said …
– *How long do I still have to wait?*	– Waving the arms and speaking with a raised voice
	– Whispering and looking away
	– Standing with the hands on the hips
	– Whiny–voiced
	– With clenched fist
	– …

3.3.2 Cultural Differences

3.3.2.1 Contextualisation

Different cultures may have rather different ideas of what kind of verbal communication is appropriate. Three areas where this is especially relevant in medical consultations are contextualisation, metaphorical language and norms about honesty. These areas are in some ways parallel to the use of understandable, respectful and honest language discussed above.

Different cultures have different norms about **how much** information should be made explicit in words and how much information should be communicated nonverbally (Hall 2004; DiMatteo et al. 1986).

- In **low-context cultures**, messages are clearly verbalised: the important ideas in a message are put in words, and it is generally regarded to be the responsibility of the speaker to make that message clear to the listener. The content of verbal communication is what is important in both conveying information and building rapport or trust.
- In **high-context cultures**, a lot of information is communicated nonverbally and through other aspects of the context. The most important information often lies in facial expressions, silence or other features of the environment. Much of what is communicated is implicit rather than explicit. For people coming from high-context cultures, nonverbal communication is important when conveying information as well as building rapport or trust.

Without wanting to stereotype, examples of lower-context cultures are Australian, New Zealand, German, English, Irish and Scandinavian. Higher-context cultures are, among others, African, Arab, French, Indian and Vietnamese.

When people with these different backgrounds communicate, misunderstandings and communication problems are possible. Someone from a high-context culture is likely to experience someone from a low-context culture as overly talkative and perhaps rude. Someone from a low-context culture might think that the person from a high-context culture is quiet, and perhaps even stand-offish. For someone from a high-context culture, a negative facial expression or lack of enthusiasm may be enough to communicate that they do not want to discuss an issue further. However, for someone from a low-context culture, such a change of subject or end of discussion may need to be stated in words before it is understood.

While talking to patients, it is helpful to understand whether they come from a high- or low-context culture. With high-context patients, pay particular attention to your nonverbal communication, including facial expressions, body posture and distance and tone of voice. With patients coming from a low-context culture try to make your verbal language as clear and explicit as possible—while remembering that patients will take you at your word. (And thus, may remind you of your words later on: 'But you told me it wouldn't hurt.')

- **Strategies**
  - Determine whether your patients are from a high- or low-context culture. Observe them attentively and listen to them carefully (see *Active Listening* Sect. 3.1).
  - If it appears that a patient comes from a high-context culture, pay particular attention to your nonverbal communication, including facial expressions, body position and distance and tone of voice.
  - If it appears that a patient comes from a low-context culture, try to make your verbal language as clear and explicit as possible.

3.3.2.2 Nonverbal Communication

Different cultures have different ideas about what kinds of nonverbal communication are appropriate in what kinds of situations. The same nonverbal behaviour can also have different meanings for people from different cultural backgrounds. The gesture of nodding, for example, can mean 'yes' or 'no' (there are some nice examples of how to nod, say 'yes', or acknowledge someone's presence on YouTube). Also hand gestures can be interpreted differently depending on where you come from. Because of this, it is important to pay attention to your own nonverbal behaviour in your interactions with patients and to keep an open mind about others' nonverbal behaviour. It can also be helpful to learn about what kind of nonverbal behaviours are and are not considered appropriate and acceptable in the country or culture you are working in. However, it is also important to avoid overgeneralising—that is, assuming that the same general beliefs apply to every individual in a culture. Moreover, as quoted in Chap. 1, patients want to be recognised as individuals:

Instead of thinking ...	Think ...
A Muslim woman wearing a headscarf is: – Conservative – Dependent on her husband ...	This woman may be: – Emancipated – A successful businesswoman – Single ... and has made a conscious decision to be wearing a headscarf

3.3.3 Forms of Nonverbal Communication

3.3.3.1 Appearance and Dress

Our appearance—which includes elements like the clothes we wear, our haircut and our posture—says a lot about us. It can be a **signal** of what national, social or professional groups we belong to. Some people may have strong reactions to these signals. Thus, it is vital to be aware that your appearance is important to your patients and that it can contribute to their impressions of you and the quality of your communication with them:

As a doctor, wearing a ...	You ...
– White coat	→ Communicates your identity as a doctor → May make people feel insecure because of the power and status this position gives you
– 'Normal' clothes	→ May confuse patients (who expect doctors to dress in a particular way) → May alienate patients

Different cultures have different norms and ideas about what is appropriate in terms of appearance and dress. What is acceptable in one culture may be seen as offensive in another. Thus, when working in a foreign country or culture, it is important to be aware of local dress codes and standards for appearance. It is also important to keep in mind that your patients may have different ideas than you do of what appropriate dress is.

- **Strategies** which will work in all contexts:
    - Try to keep an open mind about others' appearances.
    - Try to not to judge people too quickly.

3.3.3.2 Body Language: Posture, Proxemics and Haptics

The way you use your body can also say a lot about you. Such **body language** (also called kinesics) includes the way you hold yourself (posture), how much physical distance you put between yourself and other people (proxemics) and how you use touch (haptics). Norms and standards for body language often differ from person to person and from culture to culture. Someone who prefers subtle and discrete body language may be bothered or put off by a speaker with very expressive body language. On the other hand, someone who prefers expressive body language may think that someone using more subtle body language is disengaged or uninterested.

Different people and different cultures also have different ideas about **personal space** and appropriate physical distance. Some patients may feel anxious or stressed if the doctor is sitting too close to them. Others might have the impression that the doctor is uninterested in them or cold-hearted if the doctor keeps a greater distance than patients expect. Such impressions can also be affected by the size of the consultation room, or the arrangement of furniture in it.

Ideas of appropriate physical distance may also depend on **gender**. In cross-gender consultations, patients and doctors often maintain a larger physical distance than they do in same-gender consultations.

Whether and how it is appropriate to **touch** patients may be complicated and highly sensitive. Different cultures have different ideas about where and how it appropriate to touch others:

> Touching another person's head is considered to be offensive in some countries of the Middle East and Asia. (The Provider's Guide to Quality and Culture)

Generally, touching your patients is a routine part of physical examinations (see Sect. 4.3), and as such cannot be avoided. However, whether it is appropriate to touch patients during other parts of your interaction—such as whether it is appropriate to put your hand on a patient's arm when delivering bad news—depends from patient to patient. In some cultures, such as those of Eastern Europe, it is common to touch patients to comfort them. In other countries, however, this may not be common at all, particularly when the doctor and patient are different genders.

Generally, it is a good idea to pay attention to your patients' body language and respond to what this says to you in a way that helps the patient feel as comfortable as possible.

- **Strategies**
  - Ask yourself: Do they seem comfortable? Are they at their ease? Do they approach you or are they looking for more distance? Are they folding their arms?
  - Try to follow or match your patients' behaviour in terms of posture, physical distance and level of touch, to the extent possible.
  - If you are not sure whether your behaviour is appropriate, you can always ask:

> – *Is it okay if I hold your hand?*
> – *Would you like a hug?*
> – *Would you feel better if there was a larger distance between us?*

3.3.3.3 Eye Contact

In the Western world, eye contact usually communicates **interest** and **attention** and is an important component of active listening (see Sect. 3.1). Eye contact generally gives patients the impression that you are concentrating on them and what they are telling you. Avoiding eye contact, looking away or staring at the ground is often considered impolite and can be interpreted as a sign of disinterest or dishonesty.

However, it is important to be aware that in some cultures, direct eye contact may be seen as **rude** or **threatening**:

In Asian or African cultures …	May mean that …
– Directly looking at a person	→ You are staring at them → You are violating their privacy

In the Western world, eye contact is considered particularly important when doctors and patients are discussing a **diagnosis** and planning next steps for treatment or **management** of patients' medical problems. Here, maintaining direct eye contact can help you be sure that patients understand what you are saying. However, as discussed above, this may make some people uncomfortable.

- **Strategies**
  - As with other types of nonverbal behaviour, it is generally best to **monitor** your patients' level of comfort and adapt your own behaviour to what makes them the most comfortable.
  - For some, this will mean looking them in the eye; for others, it may mean directing your gaze elsewhere.
  - If you cannot avoid doing something that makes your patient uncomfortable, explain the reason for your behaviour:

When you …	You …
– Work on the computer – Take notes – Consult a file …	→ Talk to your patient → Look up once in a while → Explain what you are doing and why → Make sure the patient does not feel abandoned

3.3.3.4 Tone and Use of Voice

Your voice, and the way you use your voice, carries a lot of **information** about who you are. It also affects the way that people interpret and understand what you say, as well as the impressions that they form of you. Tone and use of voice includes how quickly or slowly you speak, how clearly you articulate your words, how much you modulate your voice (that is, speaking in a monotone versus a lot of changes in pitch) and how loud you speak, among other factors. A recent study of surgeons found that doctors' tone of voice could predict the number of malpractice claims they had (Ambady et al. 2002). Thus, it is important to be aware of how you are using your voice (see also White et al. 1994):

If your voice sounds …	Try to …
– Strident (loud and hard)	→ Breath from the diaphragm (avoid shallow breathing)
– Dry and scratchy	→ Drink enough water when you talk all day long
	→ Sit up straight (posture affects breathing)
– Tired	→ Use gestures to make your voice sound energetic (especially when you are tired)
	→ Smiling may also help
– High–pitched	→ Practise speaking at a slightly lower pitch to enhance your credibility

Tone and use of voice can communicate your level of interest, engagement and knowledge. It can affect how much patients think you care and how competent they think you are (Lown 1999). It often affects the level of trust. Using the right tone of voice can help patients feel more **comfortable** and less anxious and improve the overall quality and effectiveness of your communication with them.

Tone and use of voice becomes increasingly important when you are not in **face-to-face** contact with your patient (see Sect. 5.4).

Different people, and different cultures, may have different **expectations** for what kind of quality of voice is appropriate. Some patients may want and expect you to speak slowly and clearly, while others might feel patronised by this kind of speech and would prefer you speak to them more quickly.

- **Strategies**
  - When talking to your patients, pay attention to their responses to the way you are using your voice.
  - As with other nonverbals, try to adapt your voice to what your patients seem to be most comfortable with.
  - Be flexible and adaptable; this is an important part of being an effective communicator.

3.3.3.5 Silence

Silence can also carry a lot of **meaning**, and different cultures have different ideas of how appropriate or acceptable silence is. In some cultures, and to some individual people, periods of silence are accepted: they are often seen as a sign that someone is thinking about how best to respond. In other cultures, and to other people, however, silence is seen as something suspicious or uncomfortable that should be filled in as quickly as possible.

Different cultures also have different beliefs about how **appropriate** it is to interrupt another person, or to have two people speaking at once. In Nordic countries, interruptions and simultaneous speech are generally seen as disrespectful. However, in southern European countries, interruptions are often seen as a sign on enthusiasm and involvement.

Doctors' use of silence can affect the **quality of** their **communication** with patients. Sometimes, being silent for a short period can be an effective way to encourage patients to continue speaking. In these cases, being silent may help you learn important pieces of information you would not have found out otherwise. On the other hand, such silences may make some patients uncomfortable and cause them to question your competence (i.e. wondering why you, as the medical authority, are not telling them what you think, or what to do). If you feel that patients are confused or troubled by silences in the conversation, you can explain to them that you want them to have all the time they need to remember every important detail they want to tell you.

- **Strategies**
  - As suggested with other kinds of nonverbal behaviour, pay attention to your patients' reactions to your use of silence and how they use silence themselves.
  - Some patients may need more time to react to what you have said (resulting in silence while they prepare themselves). Others may be uncomfortable with silence and try to avoid it.
  - Try to adapt your own use of silence to what makes patients most comfortable and what helps make the consultation as effective as possible.

3.4 Building Rapport

For a medical consultation to be effective and successful, there needs to be a **good relationship** between you and your patients (Sect. 3.4.2.1), but also the rapport with your colleagues (Sect. 3.4.2.2) will have an effect on the entire medical encounter. A determining factor is the gender of the person you communicate with (Sect. 3.4.3). Here, building rapport refers to developing this relationship through the way you communicate. Building rapport is important: it helps make both communication and consultations more effective, efficient, supportive and satisfying for both medical professionals and patients (Fernández 2010).

3.4.1   Expectations

When we start a conversation with someone, we have certain expectations about what they will do and how they will communicate. The people we are talking with, in turn, have similar expectations about us. Generally, communication goes smoothly when people act in ways that are consistent with our expectations.

Communicating in a way that meets patients' desires and expectations—while also meeting your own—will help the consultation be more **satisfying** and more **effective** for you and your patients. For more on specific skills for effective listening, verbal communication and nonverbal communication, see the corresponding sections in this chapter.

Generally, patients come to the consultation with desires and expectations:

- They expect their doctors to be **competent** and knowledgeable. Patients want an expert doctor. They are coming to you because of your professional expertise.
- Patients also want their doctor to be a **sympathetic** human being (friendly and concerned about their problem(s) and well-being). They need to be able to relate to their doctor:
  - Patients want to feel respected and understood.
  - Patients want to feel that you care about them and that you will support them even when things are difficult.
  - Patients want to be taken seriously, and want to actively participate in the decision-making process.

The best way to meet patients' expectations will depend on the individual and cultural background of a patient: respect, understanding or empathy, for example, may be communicated in many different ways. As discussed above, something like touching a patient to comfort them can be customary and appropriate in some cultures, but inappropriate in others. Paying attention to your patients' behaviour and reactions is the best way to gauge what they are or are not comfortable with.

3.4.2   Professional Relationships

3.4.2.1   Doctor–Patient Relationship

Patients from different cultures may have different expectations about the **nature** of the doctor–patient relationship. These expectations will affect what kind of communication they believe is appropriate.

Generally, patients from more **egalitarian** cultures expect to be treated more like a peer. They usually want to be involved in discussions and decisions about their treatment options and related planning. They may see you more as an advisor than an all-powerful authority figure. They will expect you to provide rationales and explanations for your recommendations and may question or challenge you on your suggestions.

In contrast, patients from more **hierarchical** cultures may expect and/or prefer a more authoritarian style of interaction. They may neither expect nor want to be involved in discussing treatment options. Rather, they want to be told what is best—in their mind, you are the knowledgeable authority. Being asked to be involved in decision-making related to their treatment may make them uncomfortable or cause them to question your competence and professionalism. Similarly, behaving or speaking informally with these kinds of patients may have the same effect. Elderly patients, in particular, are often more sensitive to formality and expect a more formal relationship between doctor and patient. They will treat you with respect and use all the expected honorifics like titles and formal *you*. Patients coming from more hierarchical cultures may also be more hesitant to ask you questions, especially why questions, because such questions could be interpreted as a sign of distrust or disrespect.

- **Strategies**
  - Try to understand what expectations your patient has for their relationship with you (e.g. formal versus informal; authoritarian versus advisory).
  - Make attempts to involve your patients in discussions and decision-making (e.g. with respect to their treatment) according to their individual preferences—there is no 'one-size-fits-all' solution.
  - Be prepared for your patients to ask you questions and possibly question your decisions or recommendations.
  - If you feel unsure about how to behave, it is better to be more formal rather than informal.

3.4.2.2 Relationship with Colleagues

Although most of this book focuses on communication between doctors and patients, doctors' communication with **colleagues** is also important because their interactions with colleagues have direct consequences for both patients' health and their own professional success (Dunn and Markoff 2009; Garelick and Fagin 2004). In a study by Gasiorek and Van de Poel (2012) among mobile medical professionals ($n = 134$) and their native colleagues ($n = 52$) in five Western European countries, participants agreed on the mobile medics' additional training needs related to everyday medical language, fluency, idioms, pronunciation, humour and local dialects. Beyond this, however, assessments diverged: the mobile medics generally felt confident in their communication skills (and thought other saw them as competent), but their colleagues reported a number of concerns, including difficulties with small talk, nonverbal communication and observance of local cultural norms.

A particularly important professional relationship is the one between doctor and nurse: doctors and nurses are mutually interdependent, and often the quality of care a patient receives depends on how well they are able to communicate and work together. However, this relationship can be problematic: in a recent survey of UK nurses, almost 50 % of participants were dissatisfied with their relationships with doctors, particularly in teaching hospitals, where there was an atmosphere of competitiveness. Only 40 % felt they were consulted about clinical matters, and almost 50 % believed that doctors never read their notes.

Doctors and nurses have different relationships with **patients**, and this can have important consequences (Porter 1991). While doctors generally provide patients with information, discuss treatment options and work with patients to determine what they will do next, they often do not spend as much time with patients as nurses do. Spending this time with patients, nurses often provide more emotional support, have longer conversations with them and generally get to know them better. Sometimes, nurses may come to disagree with doctors' recommendations or treatment plans. In these cases, nurses often would like to have their opinions heard. However, often, doctors do not ask them for their opinion, or take their views into consideration.

The nature and quality of the relationship between doctors and nurses can differ considerably in different places and depends on a number of different factors. In some places, doctors and nurses see each other as near-peers, while in other places, doctors are generally considered to be superiors and nurses to be subordinates. The doctor–nurse relationship also depends on the education, competencies and tasks nurses and doctors each have. This may vary considerably from hospital to hospital or country to country:

Nurses from Spain and England working in German hospitals are surprised because they …	Doctors from China and Russia working in German hospitals feel indignant because they …
– Have few responsibilities – Have to do 'unskilled labour' – Cannot take blood samples from patients – Cannot take care of wound treatment → Spanish, Polish and British nurses (usually) have a university degree	– Have to take blood samples from patients – Feel the German nurses should take care of this → German nurses do not have a university degree

As with doctor–patient relationships, whether a person comes from a more egalitarian or more hierarchical culture can affect their expectations for doctor–nurse communication.

In more **hierarchical** societies, it is rare for a nurse (or a paramedic) to question a doctor's expertise. However, in more **egalitarian** cultures, it is more common for nurses or other subordinates to question doctors' decisions, which could be considered as a sign of disrespect by doctors used to a more hierarchical relationship between doctors and nurses. Nurses used to a more egalitarian doctor–patient relationship may feel offended and even start questioning the doctors' expertise if the doctors do not answer their questions or appear to take them seriously.

In the Western world, we are seeing the relationship between doctors and nurses shifting. In general, nurses are being given more responsibility, and the social and professional disparity between doctors and nurses is decreasing. This is partially due to the introduction of clinical nurse specialists and nurse consultants, among other reasons.

- **Strategies**
  - Try to find out how the hierarchy in your hospital and hospital unit is structured by observing your colleagues. Are they calling each other with their first names or their family names? Do they use titles? What is the nature of the doctor–nurse relationship? Does it seem to be hierarchical or more egalitarian? Is it common that nurses talk with doctors about their decisions or not?

- Accept existing rules of hierarchy even though they seem strange to you. If possible, try to discuss them with some colleagues of yours you like or appreciate. Tell them about your experiences and opinions without imposing on them.
- If you are used to a more hierarchical doctor–nurse relationship and a nurse is asking for a rationale, do not take it personally: treat it as an opportunity to teach.
- Make sure you know the names of all the nurses on the unit and introduce yourself to new arrivals.
- Seek informal opportunities to meet with nurses, and seek their input on clinical matters when appropriate.
- When giving instructions make sure that you address them to the senior nurse who will delegate to other nurses if necessary.

3.4.3   Communication and Gender

Gender is an important factor to consider when thinking about building rapport through communication (Butler 1993; West 1990). Men and women often use language differently and indeed communicate differently. Some researchers have suggested that we can think of gender as a **culture**, and so many of the same ideas that apply to intercultural communication can also be applied to communication between men and women.

Studies on medical communication and gender have found that compared to male doctors, female doctors tend to have a more **cooperative** and **accommodative** attitude towards their patients and tend to respond more to their patients' wishes. Female doctors also tend to emphasise the status difference between doctor and patient less. Male doctors, on the other hand, tend to focus more on the objective medical problem than on their patients' concerns (and this is particularly the case when patients are women).

Generally, it is important to be aware that you or others may be using particular approaches to communication, or have particular expectations about communication, without realising it, and that these approaches and expectations may be related to gender. As with all cultural differences, try to understand the **specific needs** of your patients, and respond to those. Try yourself to be as flexible as possible in your use of language and in your communication more generally. Make an effort to do what makes your patients feel most comfortable rather than force your own ideas or expectations on to your patients.

3.5   Summary

In this chapter, we highlighted communication skills that you can use across all stages of the consultation. We focused on how active listening skills facilitate, direct and structure your interaction with others, what makes verbal and nonverbal communication appropriate and how the way you communicate builds rapport between you and your patients.

Main Points

- Good listening is active listening.
- Active listening is attentive and responsive.
- Active listening involves skills that help facilitate, direct and structure your interaction.
- How you say something can be as important as what you say.
- Medical language use is right if it is understandable, respectful and honest.
- The focus of our verbal communication is generally the content of our messages.
- Our attitudes about what we say are often communicated through our nonverbal behaviour.
- In most cases, our nonverbal behaviour supports our verbal behaviour.
- If the two contradict each other, people tend to believe the nonverbal message more than the verbal message.
- Keep an open mind about others' nonverbal behaviour.
- Our appearance can be a signal of what national, social or professional groups we belong to.
- Norms and standards for body language often differ from person to person and from culture to culture.
- Eye contact usually communicates interest and attention.
- Tone of voice carries information about who you are.
- The use of silence can affect the quality of your communication with patients.

Building rapport through effective communication is important for developing a good working relationship with your patients and your colleagues.

Additional Reading

→ Active Listening

Fassaert T, Van Dulmen S, Schellevis F, Bensing J (2007) Active listening in medical consultations: Development of the Active Listening Observation Scale (ALOS-global). Patient Educ Couns 68 (3):258–264

→ Appropriate Verbal Communication

Pendleton D et al. (2007) The new consultation. Developing doctor-patient communication. Oxford University Press, Oxford

Silverman J et al. (2006) Skills for communicating with patients. Radcliffe Publishing, Oxford/San Francisco

Tate P (2007) The doctor's communication handbook. Radcliffe Publishing, Oxford/ Seattle

→ Doctor-Doctor/Nurse Relationship

Dunn AS, Markoff B (2009) Physician-physician communication: what's the hang-up? J General Intern Med 24:437–439

Garelick A, Fagin L (2004) Doctor to doctor: getting on with colleagues. Adv Psychiat Treat 10:225–232

Iedema R (ed.) (2007) The discourse of hospital communication. Tracing complexities in contemporary health care organizations. Palgrave Macmillan, Houndmills/New York

Lumma-Sellenthin A (2009) Talking with patients and peers: medical students' difficulties with learning communication skills. Med Teach 31:528–534

→ Doctor-Patient Relationship

Roter DL, Hall JA (2006) Doctors talking with patients/patients talking with doctors: improving communication in medical visits. Praeger, Westport

Sudore RL, Landefeld CS, Pérez-Stable EJ, Bibbins-Domingo K, Williams, BA, Schillinger D (2009) Unraveling the relationship between literacy, language proficiency, and patient–physician communication. Patient Couns Educ 75:398–402

Travaline JM (2005) Patient-physician communication: why and how. JAOA 1:13–18

→ Gender

Butler J (1993) Bodies that matter: on the discursive limits of "sex". Routledge, New York

West C (1990) Not just doctors' orders: directive-response-sequences in patients' visits to women and men physicians. Discourse Soc 13:843–851

→ Metaphors

Ruthrof H (2000) The body in language. Cassell, London/New York

Yu N (2009) The Chinese HEART in a cognitive perspective: culture, body and language. Mouton de Gruyter, Berlin/New York

→ Nonverbal Communication

Beattie G (2003) Visible thought. The new psychology of body language. Hove, Routledge

Fernández EI (2010) Verbal and nonverbal concomitants of rapport in health care encounters: implications for interpreters. J Specialised Transl 14:216–228.

Watzlawick P, Beavin Bavelas J, Jackson DD (2011) Pragmatics of human communication. WW Norton & Company, New York

→ Tone of Voice

Ambady N, LaPlante D, Nguyen T, Rosenthal R, Chaumeton N, Levinson W (2002) Surgeon's tone of voice: a clue to malpractice history. Surgery 132:5–9

DiMatteo MR, Hays RD, Prince LM (1986) Relationship of physicians' nonverbal communication skills to patient satisfaction, appointment compliance and physician workload. Health Psych 5:581–594

References

Ambady N, LaPlante D, Nguyen T, Rosenthal R, Chaumeton N, Levinson W (2002) Surgeon's tone of voice: a clue to malpractice history. Surgery 132:5–9

Beattie G (2003) Visible thought: the new psychology of body language. Routledge, Hove

Butler J (1993) Bodies that matter: on the discursive limits of "Sex". Routledge, New York

DiMatteo MR, Hays RD, Prince LM (1986) Relationship of physicians' nonverbal communication skills to patient satisfaction, appointment compliance and physician workload. Heal Psychol 5:581–594

Dunn, AS & Markoff B (2009) Physician–physician communication: What's the hang-up? Journal of General Internal Medicine, 24:437–439

Fassaert T, Van Dulmen S, Schellevis F, Bensing J (2007) Active listening in medical consultations: development of the active listening observation scale (ALOS-global). Patient Educ Couns 68(3):258–264

Fernández EI (2010) Verbal and nonverbal concomitants of rapport in health care encounters: implications for interpreters. J Spec Transl 14:216–228

Garelick A, Fagin L (2004) Doctor to doctor: getting on with colleagues. Adv Psychiatr Treat 10:225–232

Gasiorek J, Van de Poel K (2012) Divergent perspectives on language-discordant mobile medical professionals' communication with colleagues: an exploratory study. J Appl Commun Res 1–16. doi:10.1080/00909882.2012.712708

Hall P, Keely E, Dojeiji S, Byszewski A & Marks M (2004) Communication skills, cultural challenges and individual support: Challenges of international medical graduates in a Canadian healthcare environment. Medical Teacher, 26:120–125.

Lown B (1999) The lost art of healing: practising compassion in medicine. Ballantine Books, New York

Makoni S (1998) Conflict and control in intercultural communication: a case study of compliance-gaining strategies in interactions between black nurses and white residents in a nursing home in Cape Town, South Africa. Multilingua 17:227–248

Pendleton D et al (2007) The new consultation: developing doctor-patient communication. Oxford University Press, Oxford

Porter S (1991) A particular observation study of power relations between nurses and doctors in a general hospital. J Adv Nurs 16:728–735

Ruthrof H (2000) The body in language. Cassell, London/New York

Silverman JD, Kurtz SM, Draper J (2006) Skills for communicating with patients. Radcliffe Publishing, Oxford/San Francisco

Tate P (2007) The doctor's communication handbook. Radcliffe Publishing, Oxford/Seattle

Watzlawick P, Beavin Bavelas J, Jackson DD (2011) Pragmatics of human communication. WW Norton & Company, New York

West C (1990) Not just doctors' orders: directive-response-sequences in patients' visits to women and men physicians. Discourse Soc 13:843–851

White J, Levinson W, Roter D (1994) "Oh, by the way…" the closing moments of the medical visit. J Gen Intern Med 9:24–28

Wiseman RL (1995) Intercultural communication theory. Sage Publications, Thousand Oaks/London/New Delhi

Witte K, Morrison K (1995) Intercultural and cross-cultural health communication. Understanding people and motivating healthy behaviours. In: Wiseman RL (ed) Intercultural communication theory. Sage Publications, Thousand Oaks/London/New Delhi

Yu N (2009) The Chinese HEART in a cognitive perspective: culture, body and language. Mouton de Gruyter, Berlin/New York

Communication Skills Specific to the Consultation

4

Contents

The table of contents of this chapter follows the timeline of the consultation:

K. Van de Poel et al., *Communication Skills for Foreign and Mobile Medical Professionals*,
DOI 10.1007/978-3-642-35112-9_4, © Springer-Verlag Berlin Heidelberg 2013

What to Expect in This Chapter

In this chapter, we discuss communication skills and strategies used at specific points during the consultation. In doing so, we go through the consultation time-line introduced in Chap. 2 in greater detail, providing specific advice for different stages and parts of the consultation (see also Bickley 2007; Bickley and Szilagiy 2007; Kurtz et al. 2003; 2006; Pendleton et al. 2007; Prabhu and Bickley 2007; Silverman et al. 2006; Tate 2007).

Following the **opening of the consultation,** we will first address the topic of **medical history** or anamnesis, when listening is the focus. This first half of the consultation is usually completed with a **physical examination**. The second half of the consultation is focused on explaining and generally has two parts: (1) **explaining** the diagnosis and (2) agreeing on the **management plan** that follows from this diagnosis. Successful listening and explaining allow for a proper **closing** of the session.

We will discuss the following five consultation components:

- Opening the session
- Information gathering
- The physical examination
- Explaining and planning
- Closing the session

4.1 Initiating the Session

Everything you do from the moment you walk in the examination room contributes to building rapport with your patient. The way you greet the patient, particularly if you are meeting them for the first time, sets the tone for future communication and interaction. You want your patients to trust you, both emotionally and profession-ally, and so it is important to start consultations in a way that facilitates this.

As discussed above, patients have expectations of their doctors: they expect their doctor to be both competent and considerate (Bonvicini et al. 2009; Pendleton 1983).

- Being **competent** means that you have the medical knowledge and skills neces-sary to help them.
- Being **considerate** means that you have the interpersonal communication skills to make them feel comfortable and you care about them and their well-being. Patients want to feel supported and understood as people, not just seen as a set of medical problems to be solved.

4.1.1 Greeting and Establishing Rapport

When you walk in the room and greet your patients, they form first impressions of you. First impressions are powerful and can be difficult to change once they are established. Although what you say matters, a large part of first impressions are based on nonverbal, rather than verbal, behaviour. Thus, it is particularly important to be aware of your nonverbal behaviour when greeting the patient at the start of the consultation (Makoul et al. 2007).

4.1.2   Strategies for Greeting the Patient and Establishing Rapport

The following are useful strategies for greeting the patient and establishing rapport:
• Prepare yourself to be in a good mood (Sect. 4.1.2.1)
• Be ready to give full attention to the patient (Sect. 4.1.2.2)
• Have the consultation room prepared (Sect. 4.1.2.3)
• Address potential problems (Sect. 4.1.2.4)
• Greet the patient (Sect. 4.1.2.5)
• Be aware of your nonverbal behaviour (Sect. 4.1.2.6)
• Be aware of your verbal behaviour (Sect. 4.1.2.7)
• Be aware of names and titles (Sect. 4.1.2.8)
Sect. 4.1.2.9 contains some pointers for nonnative speakers.

4.1.2.1   Prepare Yourself to Be in a Good Mood
Your nonverbal behaviour very often reflects your mood, whether you realise it or not. It is best to do everything you can to make sure that you are in a good (positive) mood when you go to see your patient.
• Prepare yourself **mentally**. Patients come to see you because they believe you can help them. Reminding yourself of patients' expectations (see above) can also help you mentally prepare for meeting them.
• Make sure that you are **physically** comfortable. This will help you be in a good mood. If you are hungry, eat a small snack before meeting the patient. If you are thirsty, drink some water. If you are feeling tired, consider having a coffee or stretching to wake yourself up.

4.1.2.2   Be Ready to Give Full Attention to the Patient
During the consultation, you want to be able to focus your full attention on the patient. To make sure you are ready to do this:
• Complete or put aside your previous task.
• Review any relevant notes, computer records or related case information before going to see the patient.
Reviewing things ahead of time helps you avoid unnecessary hurry or distraction in the patient's presence. This allows you to concentrate your full attention on the patient as a person when you greet them and throughout the course of the consultation.

4.1.2.3   Have the Consultation Room Prepared
To maintain the **professional** nature of the consultation:
• Plan to keep the doors closed.
• Make any arrangements necessary to be sure you will not be disturbed by phone calls or other avoidable interruptions during the consultation.

- If for some reason it is not possible to do the consultation in a private space, reassure the patient that they have your full attention.
- Be aware that these circumstances may inhibit or distract the patient to the point of giving inaccurate or incomplete information.
- Explain or apologise for anything that may disrupt patient's expectations about the consultation (see the next section).

4.1.2.4 Address Potential Problems

To maintain the professional character of the whole encounter:

- **Inform** patients if you will be late. Most patients will be much less bothered by waiting if they know that you are late. You can ask the secretary or nurse to inform them.
- When you arrive, **apologise** for being late.
- Apologise for any other external circumstance that may interfere with the professional character of the consultation, such as construction in the hospital, a new administrative or records system and a lack of privacy due to the design or configuration of examination rooms.

4.1.2.5 Greet the Patient

How you greet patients strongly influences their first impression of you. To make this impression as positive as possible:

- Greet patients individually, by name, when you first meet them, either in the waiting room or in the consultation room.
- Mind that in some cultures women keep their last name when married, for example, in Belgium as opposed to the Netherlands.
- Address children directly and take them seriously.
- If applicable, stand up and walk towards a patient when they enter the room.
- Greet patients while they are fully dressed.
- Mind that in some cultures people will avert their eyes when speaking to you as a sign of respect.

4.1.2.6 Be Aware of Your Nonverbal Behaviour

As discussed in Chap. 3, patients quickly form impressions of you based largely on your nonverbal behaviour. Nonverbal behaviour that helps you make a positive impression includes:

- Smiling
- Making eye contact
- Shaking hands (if customary in your hospital or medical practice)
- Showing enthusiasm and curiosity for the coming encounter in your body language
- Avoiding signs of being in a hurry
- Avoiding signs of disinterest
- Avoiding signs of unease like shifting your eyes away from the patient
- Avoiding signs of arrogance

4.1.2.7 Be Aware of Your Verbal Behaviour

Your verbal behaviour—that is, the language you use and the words you choose—also contributes to patients' impressions of you. To make a positive impression:

- Invite patients to sit down and/or make themselves comfortable:

> – *Please sit down.*
> – *Please, take a chair.*

Start the consultation only when patients are comfortably seated.

- Apologise when you are late. A patient wants to feel recognised and acknowledged. You cannot expect them to know what is going on behind the scenes.
- Take some time—if appropriate—for some general or social questions or remarks to make patients feel at ease. In case you know your patient reasonably well, some reference to a shared topic of interest is possible:

> – *So nice to see you again. Everything all right with the children/the dog …?*

- Make eye contact: look the person you are speaking to in the eye. This makes for more meaningful conversation.
- Gap-filling: if necessary (in case you have to wait for some information or a procedure to start), prepare a few remarks of general interest (e.g. on current events). Make sure to keep up to date:

> – *The weather isn't very nice today.*
> – *Did you get here easily with all the roadworks going on?*

- Some consider it unprofessional to spend a lot of time on small talk at the beginning of the consultation (Maynard and Hudak 2008). Announce that you will make time for some social chat at a later stage of the consultation:

> – *Let's first see what I can do for you and have a chat afterwards.*

- Name, explain and apologise for any inconveniences or other circumstances that may interfere with the consultation:

> – *I hope you didn't have to wait too long with the new registration system.*

4.1.2.8 Be Aware of Names and Titles

- **Patient's Name**

  Make sure you know patients' first and last name before greeting them. When first meeting a patient, it is best to use a title and their last name. If patients would like you to use their first name, they will let you know (or you can ask). Here, it is better to be too formal than too informal. Some patients may feel that using their first name is disrespectful or patronising.

- **Doctor's Name**

  Introduce yourself as appropriate. If you are replacing someone or have been called in for a particular reason, explain your role to the patient.

Pronounce your own name clearly and slowly. If needed show your badge or letterhead/seal while saying your name.

4.1.2.9 When You Are Not a Native Speaker

- **First Impressions**

  Sometimes, openly acknowledging that you are not a native speaker of the language can help set expectations appropriately and thus facilitate communication. However, because some patients might see this as a problem, or worry that this will affect the quality of the consultation, it is best to focus any discussion of this topic on your desire to facilitate communication:

> – *I am new on the team here. If you have any problem understanding what I say, please let me know.*

- **Pronunciation**

  If the patient is new to you, check that you have the correct patient file or chart in front of you (or on screen). This is especially important when the pronunciation of the patient's name is unfamiliar to you (ask a colleague in advance).

- **Intonation**

  Use a friendly inviting intonation when checking the patient's name to call them from the waiting room or when greeting the patient and inviting them to take a seat.

4.2 Information Gathering

Information gathering consists of three parts:

- Initiating information gathering: the intake (Sect. 4.2.1)
- Exploring patient's biomedical problem(s) and context (Sect. 4.2.2)
- Closing information gathering (Sect. 4.2.3)

4.2.1 Initiating Information Gathering

Within the initial stage of information gathering, the following components can be distinguished:
- Patients' narratives (Sect. 4.2.1.1)
- Exploring the patient's perspective (Sect. 4.2.1.2)
- Agenda screening (Sect. 4.2.1.3)
- Agenda setting (Sect. 4.2.1.4)

4.2.1.1 Patients' Narratives
Patients' narratives are the stories as told by patients in their own words about the problems they are experiencing. This generally takes the form of a story, told chronologically from when the problem first started to the present. Patients' narratives are an important source of information about patients' medical issues, but how you handle them also affects patients' impressions of you and how much trust and confidence they place in you later. We will first discuss the **importance** of the patient's narratives for all implied, and then we will focus on how to **elicit** the narrative and how to **actively listen** to it.

- **Importance of Patient's Narrative for the Doctor**
It is usually a good idea to open the consultation by letting the patient tell their narrative without interruption. This is because:
  - Patients and only patients know the **reason**(s) why they have come to see you. Therefore, it is important to let them explain their agenda first, before trying to follow your own. The natural way to do this is to let the patient speak first. Patients do not come with a single symptom. Rather, they come with their ideas about their symptom(s), their concerns caused by the symptom and their hopes and expectations for treatment. If you start on your biomedical agenda (asking specific questions about the nature of their symptoms) too soon, you may never discover what they really think and feel about their symptoms and situation, what worries them or what their individual expectations are.
  - You may gain much more valuable information by withholding **judgment** for just 1 or 2 min while patients tell their stories. A patient's opening narrative may tell you all the information you need to make the diagnosis. Starting down a path of clinical reasoning prematurely is potentially dangerous as it could lead to misdiagnosis. It is much better to first listen and then diagnose.
- **Importance of Their Narrative for the Patients**
Being able and allowed to tell their own story—and having that story listened to—at the start of the consultation is also important to patients. Specifically:
  - It **reassures** patients that their concerns are being taken seriously and that you are a competent and caring professional.
  - It allows and encourages patients to share information that is important to your ability to make a proper diagnosis.

- **Eliciting Patient's Opening Narrative**
  After greeting the patient, your main communicative goal is to elicit the patient's opening narrative. In other words, focus your communication on encouraging and allowing patients to share their story. Specifically:
  - Your opening question cannot be open enough. Give the patient the freedom to talk about whatever they feel is important:

Invite the patient with …	The standard …
– *Well, now, how can I help you?*	→ *What can I do for you?*
– *Well. What brings you here today?*	
with a friendly smile and a questioning raised eyebrow.	may be perceived as asking for a concrete answer.

  - If the patient answers with just a short statement, ask questions that more specifically target the narrative:

  - *Could you tell something about it?*
  - *Could you perhaps tell your story about it?*

  - Keep your body language and other nonverbal behaviour open and friendly, communicating interest and engagement.
- **Listening to Patient's Opening Narrative**
  Following your opening question(s), listen and only listen while patients share their narratives. This may be more difficult than it sounds, because it is natural—and indeed, sometimes automatic—to start making a working diagnosis or theory while the patients are still telling their story (and sometimes even before). Try to resist that urge and listen to the patient's entire story before drawing conclusions.
  During patient's opening narrative (as during any later narrative), do your best to engage in active listening (see Sect. 3.1) and related strategies and skills. It is important to be aware that some facilitative strategies such as **repetition** (echoing) and **paraphrasing**, which can be very helpful later in the consultation, may actually be counterproductive at this stage because they can interrupt the flow of the patient's story. However, if a patient is very hesitant, it may help to provide more guidance and encouragement with either confirmation that you have understood (such as paraphrasing) or with additional questions. In short:
  - Let your patient talk and have your full attention on them while they are talking.
  - Do not interrupt; allow them to tell their entire story first.

- Encourage your patient to continue by nodding, smiling and looking interested.
- Use the neutral facilitative utterances like *uh-huh, um, yes* or *I see*.
- Be involved: Actively respond to questions and directions using your body position (e.g. lean forward) to encourage the speaker and signal interest.
- Postpone making notes or computer records until the patient has completed his opening narrative.

4.2.1.2 Exploring the Patient's Perspective and Agenda

The content of the patient's opening narrative gives you insight into the patient's perspective and related agenda (see Sect. 2.3). Exploring and understanding the patient's perspective is not always easy. Patients can sometimes be unclear about their own ideas, concerns and expectations—they just know there is a problem and that they need help, but may not be able to articulate much beyond that. Additionally, some patients may first need to feel and understand that you care about them before they can tell you what is important to them.

What you learn from patients' narratives, and what this tells you about their perspective, is important not only for making a diagnosis but also for later parts of the consultation. Understanding your patients' perspective and values can help you communicate better when discussing treatment options and sharing decision-making and planning related to next steps.

In order to optimally pick up the cues, you should pay **more than superficial attention** to the patient's narrative. Further, you should **respond to the cues**, and sometimes it can be helpful to explicitly **ask** for the patient's perspective.

- **More Than Superficial Attention**

  To make sure you are getting as much information as you can from your patients' narrative, you need to truly see and hear what they are saying. This involves active listening, which requires more than just superficial attention. Some strategies to help you with this:
  - Watch the patients' **facial** expressions. Where they look and what gestures they make? Do they make eye contact?
  - Watch their posture, muscle tone and breathing. Do they look anxious, sad or angry…? Are they fidgety, relaxed or distant…?
  - Notice how their **body** language changes during different parts of the narrative. Do they sigh, shrug or look away at a particular point?
  - Notice when a chance remark of yours makes them stop and think.
  - Be aware of **inconsistencies** between verbal and nonverbal behaviour (i.e., between what they say and what they do). These can signal something that needs further exploration.
    For example: *No, I'm not depressed* while sitting with shoulders slumped and a sad expression.
  - Listen not just to what patients say but **how** they say it. Ask yourself:
    What does patient's speech tell me? What are they really saying? How are they saying it? Is their speech high pitched, too fast or too slow, changing in volume, hesitating or no longer having normal rhythm and modulation?

– Listen for what they do **not** say or when details essential to understanding are missing. Ask clarifying questions if necessary. For example:

When they say …	You might ask …
– *I feel worse.*	→ *Worse than what?* → *In what way?* → *About something?* → *About what?*

– Be aware of how concrete versus abstract patients' **descriptions** are. If patients use abstract terms that do not have a clear, concrete meaning, seek clarification, either during the narrative or later. For example:

When you hear …	Ask …
– *It's 6 months on and I'm suffering with my nerves …*	→ *What do you mean?* → *What happened?* → *What do you expect from me?*

– Be aware of generalisations. As with abstract language, try to direct the patient towards providing more concrete information:

When you hear …	Should preferably become more concrete:
– I'm **always** getting headaches.	→ OK, does that mean **every month?**

- **Responding to the Patient's Narrative**
  As discussed above (see Sect. 3.1, *Active Listening*), an important part of active listening is responding to *cues* that patients send. This first strategy involves **picking up** on verbal and nonverbal cues and then **acknowledging** and **responding** to them.
- **Picking up on cues** means recognising them in patients' verbal and nonverbal behaviour. The best way to do this is to engage in active listening.
Picking up on cues is one way to discover the patient's hidden agenda.

- **Acknowledging cues** by, for example, nodding, means showing the patient that you have seen or heard what they are trying to communicate.
- **Responding to cues** means investigating what this cue means and what it can tell you about the patient's perspective, ideas, concerns and expectations.
  - Reflecting feelings (see Sect. 3.1.2.1) can be an effective way to respond to **nonverbal** cues. This is usually done with a short question or comment checking your interpretation of what patients are feeling:

> - *My impression is that you feel sad today. ... Is that correct?*

  - The goal is to **reassure** patients and encourage them to continue talking and/ or discuss related ideas, concerns or expectations.
    A way in which to acknowledge a patient's fear:

> - *Your headaches must have scared you! Since your father had a brain tumour. I imagine you may be thinking that you could have the same illness.*

  - Echoing or paraphrasing can be effective ways to respond to **verbal** cues:

> - *Worried? ... What do you mean?*
> - *You said that you were afraid that the pain might be something serious.*
> - *What did you think it might be?*

- **Asking for the Patient's Perspective**
  You may also explicitly ask patients about their **ideas, concerns** and **expectations** (see the ICE triad as introduced in Sect. 2.3.1).
  - **Examples of questions about patient's ideas** and beliefs are:

> - *Tell me about what you think is causing it ... is happening? ... might happen?*
> - *You've obviously been giving this some thought. Could you tell me what you've been thinking?*

- **Examples of questions about patient's concerns,** needs and fears are:

> – *Is there anything worrying you?*
> – *Could you tell me how you feel about this?*
> – *How is the back pain affecting you?*
> – *How do you think the back pain will affect you?*

- **Examples of questions about patient's expectations**, hopes and wishes are:

> – *What were you hoping to get out of our meeting today?*
> – *What are you hoping I might be able to do for you?*
> – *What do you think could help you most?*

Patients' ideas, concerns and expectations are often closely tied to their **personal, social** and **occupational circumstances**. Often, learning about these circumstances can be informative:

> – *May I ask you—it may help me understand your headaches—what do you do for a living?*

Asking patients for personal and social circumstances early in the consultation shows that you are interested in them as an individual. This can also be a way to:
- Determine if psychosocial factors are causing or influencing the problem.
- Determine if the problem has effects on patients' psychological health and social functioning.

Ideally, this early discussion of patients' psychosocial lives should be limited to specific factors that are likely to be relevant to patients' perspective on their medical problem. The rest of patients' personal and social history is best postponed to the end of the information gathering phase of the consultation or to a later encounter as appropriate. Some examples:

> – *Hum, I see ... so how often do you go out eating?*
> – *Yes, right ... so how often do you go on holiday in the course of a year?*

Try to avoid being abrupt or sharp. It can help to introduce your question with a phrase such as *Hum, I see, yes, ...* or a genuine show of interest.

- **Exploring the Cultural Component of Patient's Perspective**
  In order to gain a complete picture of your patients, explore their perspective of illness and the cultural component of this perspective (Chugh et al. 1994; Kai 2003; Schouten and Meeuwesen 2006). In short:
  - Try to get to know your patients' **attitudes** towards health prevention. Find out if your patients are more present-oriented or more future-oriented and give them an impression of your understanding of effective health prevention before presenting them the possibilities they can use.
  - Ask for the patient's **expectations** for information, involvement and care:

    - *What would you like to see happen here?*

  - Ask patients if there are any **practices** in their culture that help them stay healthy (e.g. special treatment, medicine, artefacts). You have to be aware that your patients might combine their 'home' medication with your prescribed medicines which might cause negative health outcomes.
  - Ask patients for their **interpretation** of symptoms:
  - Try to avoid **stereotypes**, value judgments or a patronising tone, keeping in

    - *Do you consider this as normal/abnormal?*
    - *Which treatment alternatives do you think are/find efficient/effective?*

    mind that there is no singular concept of health and illness for a specific people or culture (see Sect. 1.2.3). Therefore, first ask questions about the patient and their family, rather than about their culture.
  - Be aware of culturally determined **cues** (nonverbal behaviour like eye contact, physical touch, body language, proximity, expression of affect and emotion) since they can be used and interpreted differently.
  - If you need to ask a **sensitive question,** first ask permission and explain why you need to ask it. Apologise if you have the impression that your patient feels offended.
  - Try to **talk** to your patient instead of giving them printed information in order to facilitate understanding. Patients with language problems and/or limited health literacy skills might not feel comfortable telling you that their language skills are not up to the level needed to work through printed materials.
- **Dealing with Emotion**
  Different people and different cultures have different ideas about how appropriate it is to express emotion. Closely related—and important to understanding patients' perspectives and narratives—people also differ in the extent to which they show or express pain (see Sect. 5.3.1).

It is important to be aware that you (and nursing staff) and your patients might have different ideas about expressions of pain and/or emotion. Try not to judge patients who are more or less expressive than others. Remember that their behaviour is influenced by their (cultural) identity and individual preferences, and try to respect it. Because you never can be sure what degree of pain or emotion your patient is experiencing, it is always a good strategy to ask for concrete details and clarification whenever possible. Emotions and experience of pain are covered in detail in Chap. 5.

4.2.1.3 Agenda Screening

Agenda screening means checking with the patients that you have heard and understood everything that they wish to discuss. Screening is important for several reasons:

- The problem the patient presents first may not actually be the most important one.
- Only patients know why they have come to see you. Screening the patient's agenda helps you make sure you have understood their reasons, which enables you to be more effective.
- If you start pursuing your own agenda too soon, you may never discover important concerns that the patient has, which you may be able to help address.
- Determining a patient's agenda early in the consultation helps you be more effective and efficient, as it may save time and help you avoid misdiagnosis and unnecessary prescriptions and referrals.

Agenda screening is as important in follow-up visits as it is in initial consultations. In this part of the consultation, it is important to be aware that the patient may not have told you their entire agenda in their opening narrative. Thus, it is important to be thorough in your screening and be prepared to find out additional, new information.

The process of agenda screening has two steps.

1. First, **summarise** what you heard and understood from patient's opening narrative about both the nature of the medical problem and the patient's perspective on it. It can be helpful to announce (signpost) that you will be confirming and summarising what you have understood up to that point:

> – *Let me summarise what I understood.*

2. Second, **ask** the patient if there is anything you have missed or if there is anything they would like to add:

> – *Is there anything else?*
> – *Has anything else been bothering you?*

Do not hesitate to check meaning and interpretation:
- Do not hesitate to ask a patient to repeat certain information in order to check that you have understood them correctly:

> – *Could you please repeat the last bit you said?*
> – *Have I understood you correctly ...?*

- If you are still unsure (because of speed, accent or the stress of the situation), invite your patient to write down a particular term or phrase.
- When this situation takes place over the phone and you feel you have missed part of the content, ask for an email confirmation of what has been said (see Sect. 5.4.1).

4.2.1.4 Agenda Setting

Agenda setting means agreeing on how to proceed next. Agenda setting naturally follows agenda screening. It is good practice to always set a formal agenda when a patient has more than one problem you need to attend to.

Agenda setting has several advantages:
- It makes the next steps (and overall organisation) of the consultation clear and explicit to you and your patient.
- Priorities can be established and negotiated.
- Setting the agenda can help you verbalise your thoughts to the patient (about how best to proceed, and otherwise).

The agenda is something that can be **negotiated** with the patient. Doing so helps the patient feel involved in the consultation process and allows you to get their consent and agreement for what is to come. To make sure the patient understands what you are doing, it can be helpful to *signpost* that you will now be agenda setting:

> – *Let me tell you how we will proceed.*

Do everything you can to use understandable, respectful and clear **language** (see above) during the process of agenda setting. Try to avoid using jargon whenever possible. It may also help to signpost when you are moving from one agenda item to the next:

> – *First, I will look at your knee to see what's wrong and what can be done. Then we will look at how to address your mobility problems.*

Thinking aloud and providing a **rationale** for each item on the agenda can help your patients better understand why you are suggesting a particular agenda or agenda item:

> – *First, I want to solve your pain problem. This will then make it much easier to make the correct plans to meanwhile cushion the effects of the pain on your living.*
> – *First, I will look at your knee to see what's wrong and what can be done. This then will make it much easier then to find 'the best way' to solve your mobility problems.*

Set **time limits** and formulate proposals. At the end, check for your patient's consent or agreement with the proposed agenda:

> – *How does that sound?*
> – *Is this all right with you?*

4.2.2 Exploring the Biomedical Perspective

Exploring the biomedical perspective of patient's problem(s)—that is, what is going on medically—is your goal and responsibility as a doctor. Having actively listened to patients' opening narrative and then screened their agenda, you have already gathered a lot of information about the biomedical aspects of their problem(s). However, you may still learn new information in the process of taking a traditional medical history, which is the primary process by which doctors explore the biomedical perspective of patients' problem(s).

In this section, we will discuss the following topics:
- Sequence of events (Sect. 4.2.2.1)
- Symptom analysis (Sect. 4.2.2.2)
- Relevant systems review (Sect. 4.2.2.3)
- Relevant background and context information (Sect. 4.2.2.4)
- General strategies to broach sensitive topics (Sect. 4.2.2.5)

4.2.2.1 Sequence of Events

The sequence of events is the **biomedical backbone** of patient's narrative(s). Patient's narratives—including their *opening narrative*—are the stories as told by the patients in their own words about any problem they are experiencing from when it first started up to the present. These stories are usually told in much the same way as they would be to a friend.

If two or more unrelated problems are the reason for the consultation, there may be more than one narrative to be elicited. When a patient has more than one reason to come to see you, you will have to clearly signpost your intention to start gathering information about the different topics. Again, the basic strategy for eliciting the narratives is by asking as **open questions** as possible.

Tips for eliciting patient's narrative(s):

- First, **signpost** the topic to be explored, for example:

> – *Let us now look at your headaches ....*

Signposting may be preceded by summarising the previous topic.

- Then, start **information gathering** with an *open question* that cannot be open enough, using a somehow curious and inviting intonation, for example:

> – *Tell me about it.*

- If appropriate, **encourage** patients to tell the story in their own words, for example:

> – *I see you are hesitating. Can you just tell me about it like you would if you were talking to a friend?*

4.2.2.2 Symptom Analysis

Symptom analysis is the process of gathering more information about patients' symptoms, usually following a patient's narrative. Following (and perhaps even during) a patient's narrative, it is likely you will have already formed a working hypothesis about the patient's condition. Having a working hypothesis based on clinical diagnostic reasoning helps you decide what questions to ask next (i.e., how to direct your anamnesis) to help you confirm or disconfirm this hypothesis. Knowing what questions you want to ask next also helps you gain information you may need to identify serious or life-threatening conditions.

During symptom analysis, you usually move gradually from **exploring** the symptom(s) to making a reliable **diagnosis**. This may involve focusing on a single symptom and system or moving between several symptoms and systems, depending on the patient's situation.

All symptoms can be classified in terms of ten different dimensions. To have a complete understanding of the nature of the patient's symptoms, you may want to ask about each of these dimensions individually.

- Character or quality:
  - *What is it like?*

- Severity or quantity:
  - *How bad is it?*
- Site or location:
  - *Where is it?*
  - *Does it radiate?*
- Timing:
  - *When did or does it start?*
  - *How long does it last?*
  - *How often does it occur?*
- Setting in which it occurs (which can suggest environmental factors that may contribute to the illness):
  - *Was that while you were at home?*
- Associated symptoms:
  - *Did you feel anything else at the same time?*
- Aggravating (and relieving) factors:
  - *Does anything make it worse?*
  - *Does anything make it better?*
  - *Does anything help?*
- Beliefs:
  - *What do you think that it is?*
- Emotional reactions:
  - *How did it make you feel?*
- Attempted therapy:
  - *Have you tried anything to treat the symptoms?*

A known memory acronym for *symptom dimensions* is **WWQQAA + B**: **W**hen (timing), **W**here (location), **Q**uality (character), **Q**uantity (severity), **A**ggravating (+setting) and alleviating factors (+therapy), **A**ssociated symptoms + **B**eliefs. Another mnemonic is **SOCRATES** (Site, Onset, Character, Radiation, Alleviating Factors, Timing, Exacerbating factors, Severity).

In symptom analysis, you nearly always use the **open-to-closed** cone of questioning, moving from open questions to focused open questions to closed questions. Some more examples:

– *Character:*	*Where do you feel the pain? Does it radiate?*
– *Aggravating factor:*	*How bad is the pain?*
– *Location:*	*Which part of your head is affected?*
– *Duration:*	*Did it start at about the same time as your dizziness?*
– *Setting:*	*What was going on when it started/ happened?*
– *Relieving factor:*	*What have you tried so far to relieve the symptoms/pain?*
– *Associated symptoms:*	*Have you noticed anything else that accompanies it?*
– *Effect of medication:*	*Did the tablets help?*

For the symptom **pain** you could ask:

– Character:	What kind of pain is it? Is it a throbbing or a cutting pain?
– Severity:	Does it wake you up at night? How often do you get them?
– Site:	Where do you get the pain? Show me exactly where you get the pain.
	Does it spread anywhere else?
– Time:	When do you get the pain? Did it come on slowly or suddenly?
	How long have you had this pain? When do they stop?
– Setting:	Does anything special bring it on? (Emotional disturbance, exercise, food, position, etc.)
– Influencing factors:	Does anything make them worse? Does anything relieve it? (Drug, exercise, food, heat, position, rest)
– Association:	Do you feel anything else wrong when it's there?

Throughout this interview, you are using the communicative skills discussed in Chap. 3 to both respond to what the patient is saying and actively structure the interview. Structuring helps keep the format and progression of the interview clear to both you and the patient. Throughout the interview, it is also helpful to use active listening skills and techniques (see Sect. 3.1).

In summary:

- **Encourage** patients to tell you the story of their symptoms and to clarify or elaborate in their own words.
- **Watch and listen** to the patient carefully, so you can respond to both verbal and nonverbal cues that they give (even though you are within a disease framework, the search of the illness frame occurs in parallel).
- Allow the patient to complete statements **without interruption**: leave space for the patient to think (and potentially continue) following pauses.
- **Facilitate** the patient's responses verbally and nonverbally using encouragement, silence, repetition and paraphrases (including interpretation).
- Try to clarify statements that are too vague or need further **elaboration**.
- Periodically **summarise** to check your own interpretation of what has been said and allow the patient to correct or to complete the information you summarise.
- Use **understandable** language and avoid jargon whenever possible; if jargon is unavoidable, apologise and then explain the jargon words you are using.

4.2.2.3 Relevant Systems Review

Following the patient's narrative and symptom analysis, you may need to review one or more other systems to obtain additional information. Reasons to do this include being sure that you are not missing a life-threatening or serious condition or gathering specific information to verify a hypothesis you have.

In a relevant system review, you nearly always use the open-to-closed cone of questioning, moving from open questions to focused open questions to closed questions.

Here, you also use the other skills and techniques of active listening for information gathering outlined above.

4.2.2.4 Background and Context Information

Following the patient's narrative, the symptom analysis and a relevant systems review, it is usually still a good idea to complete your verbal investigation by exploring the background and context of patient's problem(s). This helps you:

- Get a complete picture of the patient's symptoms and situation
- Decrease the risk of missing an important piece of information
- Extend your understanding of patient's perspective and thus improve your rapport with the patient

At this point in time, the **complete history** and the **focused history** diverge. The **complete** medical history is comprehensive, covering all aspects of patient's background. This is the type of medical interview that medical students are generally taught to perform. This type of interview is also routinely done to complete hospital medical records (which may be a cooperative process between medical students and junior staff in academic and/or teaching hospitals). The **focused** history is substantially shorter in duration and narrower in scope than complete histories. Practising doctors usually take focused histories. Generally, both types of histories follow the same communicative format—the *open-to-closed cone* of questioning—but a focused history involves much more limited closed questioning than a complete history.

The content of background and context includes information about:

- Past medical history:

> – *Have you ever had any serious illnesses in the past?*
> – *Have you ever been in a hospital for any reason?*
> – *Has there been any change in your health since your last visit?*

- Drug and allergy history:

> – *Has your doctor prescribed any medication for your condition?* (prescription)
> – *Are you taking any tablets/medication at the moment?* (factual questions)
> – *Do you always remember to take it?* (time-related questions)
> – *Do you experience any side effects?* (side effects and allergies)

- Family history:

> - *Are your parents alive and well?* (parents)
> - *Do you have any brothers and sisters (siblings)?* (relatives)
> - *Do you have any children?* (children)
> - *Are all your close relatives alive?* (family health)
> - *What was your parent's home like?*

- Personal and social history:

> - *How old are you now?* (date of birth)
> - *Do you have a partner? (What is his/her age, sex, living and working situation?)* (marital status)
> - *Are any of your children at school?* (children)
> - *Are you happy to be living on your own?* (satisfaction)
> - *Has anything changed recently?* (changes)
> - *Does your relationship make your complaint worse?* (interaction–complaint relationship)

And if necessary on the basis of the above data, the review of systems is completed.

When exploring a patient's relevant background and context information, make use of the skills and techniques for **active listening** (see Sect. 3.1). As with other types of information gathering, you will generally move from open questions first to focused open questions and then to closed questions as necessary. As in other stages of information gathering, try to:

- Watch and listen to the patient carefully, so you can respond to both verbal and nonverbal cues that they give.
- Allow the patient to complete statements without interruption: leave space for the patient to think (and potentially continue) following pauses.
- Facilitate the patient's responses verbally and nonverbally using encouragement, silence, repetition and paraphrases (including interpretation).
- Try to clarify statements that are too vague or need further elaboration.
- Periodically summarise to check your own interpretation of what has been said and allow the patient to correct or to complete the information you summarise.
- Use understandable language and avoid jargon whenever possible; if jargon is unavoidable, apologise and then explain the jargon words you are using.

It is at this stage of the information gathering that you may have to broach **sensitive topics**. Most doctors (and patients) experience at least some discomfort with certain subjects, such as use and abuse of alcohol or drugs, sexual history, mental health and family violence. Chapter 5 contains a detailed discussion of sensitive medical topics. What follows are some general strategies.

4.2.2.5 General Strategies for Broaching Sensitive Topics

When exploring background and context of a medical problem, sensitive topics may come up. When discussing sensitive topics, you use many of the same communication strategies and skills that you do discussing other topics. However, because these topics are sensitive, it is important to be very aware of your communication and take particular care in how you ask questions and respond to what patients say.

The following are some basic principles that can help guide your response to sensitive topics:

- **Be non-judgmental.** Showing disapproval of behaviour expressed in the health history can compromise your rapport with the patient. Disapproval may be interpreted as disrespectful or even humiliating by patients. If they feel you do not respect them, this compromises your rapport with them and the effectiveness of the consultation.
  - Being non-judgmental is facilitated by focussing on what really matters for you and for the patient. Rather than focussing on what you think about their behaviour, focus on what this information helps you understand about the patient's situation.
  - Use non-judgmental language. Non-judgmental language is matter-of-fact, direct language. This means using descriptive, concrete and specific words and sentences; asking for specific data or examples; and explaining what you mean whenever necessary:

A question like …	Is obviously less judgmental and more direct and descriptive than:
– *Can you tell me about your use of alcohol?*	→ *Do you drink a lot?*

- **Explain why you need to know the sensitive information**. Giving a rationale for discussing a sensitive topic helps a patient understand why you need to discuss something that might make them (or you) uncomfortable. Providing a rationale can also be a good introduction to the sensitive topic. One way to do this is through a 'normalising' statement—that is, a statement that explains to the patient that it is normal for you to ask for this kind of information (and that is why you are asking them about it):

  – *Because abuse is common in many women's lives, I've begun to ask about it routinely.*

- **Choose an appropriate time** in the history taking to broach a sensitive topic. Your mental map of the consultation is your best guide. Strategically timing this can also help you explain why you need to gather this sensitive information.
- **Avoid potential distractions or disturbances** such as being in a hurry, being interrupted or double consultations (of, e.g. husband and wife).
- As in other phases of information gathering, use the **open-to-closed** cone of questioning and make use of the techniques of active listening for information gathering.

4.2.3 Closing Information Gathering

The medical interview is usually followed by a physical examination. Generally, however, it is good practice to do a final check to make sure that both you and the patient believe that everything important has been discussed. Try to avoid ending the information gathering abruptly. Instead, indicate to the patient that it is the end of the information gathering phase by **signposting** and **summarising** what has been discussed. If you have summarised extensively during the medical interview, this final summary may be short and introduced by:

> – *Let me see, did we discuss everything?*
> – *Let's go through everything you've been telling once more.*
> – *As I see it, … is the most important conclusion of our talk so far.*

Then, give the patient time to provide **feedback**. Patients may want to accentuate what is important to them or add something that has not yet been covered:

> – *What do you feel is the most important point to remember/do/follow up/focus on?*
> – *Would you like to add something?*

Finally, explain to the patient what will happen **next**:

> – *OK, so what we're going to do next is …*
> – *I'll just check your blood pressure.*
> – *Now I'm going to tap your arm.*
> – *What happens next is that …*

This will then automatically lead into the next phase: the physical examination.

4.3   The Physical Examination

The physical examination may not only give you insights into the presence or absence of disease but also present an opportunity to learn more about your patient. The context of the examination may make the patient want to talk about deeper fears or more serious issues.

A physical examination almost always follows verbal information gathering. As discussed above, information gathering is generally concluded by your summarising the information gathered and then giving the patient the opportunity to ask questions or give additional information.

At this point in time, patients almost always want to know what your findings are. Thus, if possible, it is worthwhile to reassure them with respect to what you have found. It is important, however, to make sure that you have gathered a sufficient amount of information before reassuring patients. If you provide reassurance too early, patients could interpret your words as dismissive or uninformed, which may lead them to believe that further tests or investigations are needed. Following appropriate reassurance, patients should be more relaxed during the physical examination. If you cannot or do not want to share your findings before completing the physical examination, explain this to that patient:

> – *I understand that you would like to know what is wrong with you, but I know this only with enough certainty after the examination. We will continue this talk then. OK?*

It is possible that the physical contact and closeness of a physical examination may make patients uncomfortable. Some patients may have deep-rooted emotions and/or norms (which may vary culturally; see Sect. 3.3.2) about the appropriateness of physical contact. You can ease or prevent some of this discomfort by providing patients with procedural and relational 'safety nets':

- The **procedural 'safety net'** involves patients knowing and understanding the examination or procedure you are carrying out and knowing what will come next.
- The **relational 'safety net'** involves your reassuring the patients that you are a professional and an expert and that you care for them and their well-being.

The two types of strategies are followed by some tips and suggestions.

If deep-rooted emotions and/or norms remain an obstacle, you may need to discuss the further proceeding of the consultation using meta-communication (see Chaps. 3 and 5). You can explicitly state what you will do or talk about next (as in signposting), or you may communicate these intentions with nonverbal signals like eye contact, facial expression or tone of voice.

4.3.1 Procedural Strategies

To make sure that patients know and understand what you will be doing during the examination (or procedure) and know what comes next:

- Briefly **explain** which parts of the body will need to be undressed and which you will be examining:

> – *Could you remove your shirt, please, so I can check your chest?*
> – *You will need to undress now, but you can cover yourself with the blanket from the waist down if you want.*

- **Signpost** each part of the examination: state what you are going to do and how what you do will feel to the patient:

> – *Now, I'm going to feel under your arms.*
> – *I'm checking your heart now.*
> – *I'm going to take some blood. You'll feel a prick.*
> – *First I'll …*

- As you move through different parts of the physical examination, continue to **inform** patients of what you are doing, what you would like them to and what they are supposed to report on:

> – *Could you tell me exactly where it hurts?*
> – *Could I ask you to show me the spot?*
> – *Would you bend your knee again?*
> – *Could you say that again please? I didn't quite understand.*
> – *Could you please speak more slowly? I didn't understand.*

- There is no better way of reassuring and taking away uncertainty than 'talking the patient through the examination'. In other words, put your patient's mind at rest by explaining what you are going to do and why you are doing it (*providing rationale*), for example:

> – *This may feel a little bit uncomfortable, but I have to do a proper scan.*

- If you need to do something that may make the patient uncomfortable, apologise. This can take the form of **reassurance** combined with **warning:**

  - *I'm sorry if this hurts a little.*
  - *This may feel a little bit uncomfortable, but it won't take long.*
  - *It shouldn't be painful, but you will be aware of a feeling of pressure.*
  - *This may hurt a little, but I'll be quick.*
  - *You may feel a bit uncomfortable.*
  - *You'll feel a jab.*
  - *I'm sorry, but you might feel a little bit of discomfort.*

- Minimise how often you ask a patient to change position and refrain from saying too much during intimate examinations in order to avoid unnecessary tension.
- Make sure (check) that your patient understands when you formulate a request.
- Instruct the patient to **relax** whenever appropriate:

  - *Try to relax.*
  - *Take a deep breath in.*

- Provide **feedback**: if the patient is doing well, provide positive feedback. If patients need to change what they are doing, provide corrective feedback:

  - *Excellent, I can hear/see/feel it perfectly now.*

- **Conclude** your examination by telling patients you are finished with the physical examination and instructing them to dress. Do not leave your patients unsure of what to do after the examination. Reassure them that they do not have to hurry, especially if they are disabled or elderly. Finally, tell patients that you will speak further after they have gotten dressed:

  - *Right, thank you very much.*
  - *You can get dressed now and then come out to me.*
  - *Don't hurry. Take your time. I need some time to make notes.*

4.3.2   Relational Strategies

To make sure your patients feel that you are a professional who cares for them and their well-being, carry out your examination in an **efficient** and **effective** way, with as little hassle as possible for the patient. Moreover, try to:

- **Talk** to the patient during the physical examination. Keeping verbal contact helps patients feel like you care about them as a person. You may talk about what you are finding or ask additional questions. However, talking a lot may create tension during intimate examinations, so be aware of when you are talking, and watch patients for cues that they are feeling uncomfortable.
- Respond to **cues** regarding your patient's needs and be sensitive to the patient's facial expressions.
- There are moments during the examination in which you have to concentrate on what you are doing and finding. Announce this so that the patient will not become insecure about the **silence**.
- Show **understanding**. Remember that patients may be feeling fear, insecurity and shame. It can be helpful to inquire whether patients have had problematic or sensitive examinations before and how they feel about them. If you know a patient has had a bad experience with an examination in the past, you can be prepared to provide them additional emotional support.
- If you need to ask an additional question following something you find, try not to make this questions sound concerned. This may unnecessarily alarm the patient.
- Keep the patient **involved** in the examination by telling what you have done, reassuring them when you have 'normal' findings and announcing (signposting) and explaining what you will be doing next.
- Do not leave your patient in a state of **uncertainty**. Share your findings if appropriate. However, avoid giving reassurance too early, as it can be interpreted as a rejection or lack of knowledge on your part, especially if the patient is convinced that more investigations are needed. A procedural remark may be appropriate:

> – *I understand that you would like to know what is wrong with you, but I can only tell with certainty after the examination. We will continue our talk afterwards. Is that OK for you?*

- Be **polite** when you ask a patient to do something and give constant reassurance by the use of *don't worry, good, fine, ….*
- After the physical examination is over, wait for patients to get dressed before continuing your discussion with them.

4.4   Explaining and Planning

Explaining and planning generally take up the second half of the consultation.
Listening is the focus of the first half of the consultation, while **explaining** is the
focus of the second half. Explaining takes two forms:
- Explaining the (differential) diagnosis–hypothesis
- Explaining and planning the management plan that follows from this
  diagnosis

Generally, arriving at a working management plan has two phases:
- Agreeing on the management plan through negotiation
- Implementing the plan by enabling the patient to adhere to the plan

In this section, we will first review communication skills that are helpful for explaining and planning generally (see Chap. 3). Then, we will focus on specific skills to
help tailor and negotiate a management plan and enable the patient to adhere to that
plan.

General skills are:
- Skills for **using appropriate language** for explaining and planning
- Skills of **active listening** during explaining and planning
  Specific skills are:
- Skills for **tailoring** explaining and planning to the individual patient
- Skills for **negotiating** the management plan
- Skills for **enabling** the patient to adhere to the management plan

4.4.1   General Communication Skills for Explaining and Planning

Appropriate language: Using appropriate and understandable language will help
make information easier for patients to understand and recall (see Sect. 3.2 for a
discussion of understandable, respectful and honest language use). In short, appropriate language is:
- **Simple** and recognisable language, possibly without any jargon, abbreviations
  and other difficult or complex words and phrases.
- **Clear** language using concrete words and phrases, rather than ambiguous
  ones.
- **Respectful** language reassuring patients that you see them as *people* who have
  personal and social needs as well as medical needs. Respectful language shows
  attention, uses descriptive words and is problem-oriented without suggesting an
  opinion or evaluation or suggesting particular intentions on the part of the
  patient.
- **Problem-oriented** language focusing on the patient's medical issue, in a way
  that is clear and understandable to them allowing for *provisional or optional
  statements* and *provides rationale*.
- **Honest** language is above all things truthful. This includes being truthful about
  the seriousness of the diagnosis, the options for treatment and their prognosis.
  Generally, honest language is also clear (not vague or ambiguous) and descriptive (non-judgmental).

Active listening. Using active listening skills described in Sect. 3.1 also help make information easier for patients to understand and recall. Specifically:

- *Chunking*—that is, breaking longer explanations into smaller, more 'digestible' chunks—can help patients better process, understand and recall longer or more complex explanations and management plans.
- *Checking* understanding or acceptance can help tell you how well a patient is understanding you. This gives you a guide as to how to proceed and lets you know if you need to clarify.
- *Structuring* chunks of information in a logical sequence can aid understanding and recall. The content of diagnosis and management plan may be extensive and complex. Outlines (mental maps) to help you structure this part of the consultation have been included in Sect. 4.4.5 below.
- *Repetition* and *summarising* both reinforce information that has been said, helping patients remember it.
- *Signposting* directs attention, which can help patients understand what is being discussed and focus on what is important.
- *Picking up and responding to verbal and nonverbal cues* help you understand how the patient is feeling, which can help you determine when it is appropriate to give advice, information or reassurance.
- *Providing a rationale* for opinions, advices, choices and investigation and treatment plans can help enhance understanding and acceptance of your suggestions and decisions.

This phase of the consultation aims for sharing understanding and decisions on management and responsibilities. Therefore, the explanation has to be well-structured. Different ways to **structure** are:

- Showing steps in an argument: *First, second, then, next, finally, lastly, ...*
  - *First, I would like to discuss the results of the tests, then we will ....*
- Adding information: *And, also, as well, in addition, besides...*
  - *In addition, the tests show that ....*
- Comparing similar things: *Similarly, in the same way, ...*
  - *In the same way, the values for ....*
- Contrasting different things: *But, however, although, (even) though, despite (the fact that), while,...*
  - *Despite low values for ... the value for ... is high.*
- Introducing an example: *For example, such as, ...*
  - *This may be the case, for example, when you go abroad.*
- Making a generalisation: *Usually, normally, in general, ...*
  - *Usually, people do not find this difficult.*
- Restating a point: *In other words, that means, namely, ...*
  - *In other words, this will not cause any problems.*
- Explaining a cause or reason: *Because, since, due to, in order to, ...*
  - *Because you have been on medication for such a long time, we would now like to suggest the following course of action.*
- Showing a result: *So, therefore, consequently, ...*
  - *Therefore, staying on this medication may be beneficial.*
- Summarising and/or concluding: *To sum up, in short, in conclusion, ...*
  - *To sum up, there is no reason for alarm.*

4.4.2 Tailoring Explanations and Plans to the Individual Patient

An effective explanation results in **shared understanding**. In other words, when you explain effectively, the patient's knowledge and expectations should be consistent with your understanding of the problem and its likely prognosis. Effective explanation of the management plan should result in both you and the patient understanding and agreeing on the patient's next steps.

To achieve this shared understanding, explanations need to be **adapted** to the patient. To do this, you need to tailor both what you are telling the patient (the content) and the way you tell it (the language, the structure, the formulation and the presentation) to the individual patient's perspective (his individual *frame of reference*). In communication theory, this is known as *accommodating* the other speaker (Giles and Gasiorek 2012). Research has shown that people generally respond positively to being accommodated: when listeners are accommodated, they evaluate both conversations and speakers more positively and generally understand the content of what is said better. The key to tailoring explaining and planning to the individual patient is to relate what you say to the patient's illness framework to previously elicited ideas, concerns, expectations, feelings and effects on life. To do this successfully, you must understand the patient's starting point. Here, you draw on everything you have learned during the information gathering phase.

In practice, one way to tailor your explanation is to make **reactive use** of the patients' own ideas, concerns, expectations and language: that is, try to use the words and ideas they have used in their narrative in your explanations to them. Doing this helps fit the information you provide in your patients' worldview and explanatory models. Referring to specific things that your patient has said also gives you the opportunity to reinforce your patients' good ideas and beliefs that are helpful to them while countering their bad and/or erroneous ideas and beliefs.

To tailor your explanation to your patient:

- Use what you have learned during the information gathering phase of the consultation to assess your patient's **starting point**: what they already know, think, feel, fear and expect; their illness framework; and their experiences, feelings and concerns:

> – *I understand that the results of the test are somewhat of a shock.*
> – *Last time everything seemed OK, but now, the lab results show that …*
> – *But, as I said, at this stage, the disease is treatable.*

- If you need **additional** information to assess a patient's starting point, ask these questions before you start extensive explaining and planning:

> – *Could you be a little more precise?*
> – *Could you expand on that?*

- Try to determine how much information the patient **wants**. This can be difficult. Generally, patients want as much information as they can absorb and understand. However, how much information this is depends on the patient. Watch for cues that help tell you whether that the patient is satisfied with what you have said or would like more detail or information:

  – *I don't know whether that makes sense?*
  – *Is there anything else that you would like to know/ask about?*

- Drawing on what you know from the information gathering phase, use and **reinforce** your patients' good ideas and those beliefs that are helpful to the outcome:

  – *The only way to treat this is indeed by an operation. It is routine surgery, we have a team of experienced surgeons here and you should be back to normal 2 months after the operation.*

- **Counter** patients' bad and erroneous beliefs. Both countering their erroneous ideas and reinforcing their good ideas help them understand their situation, which can then help them decide what they want to do:

  – *This is quite a common condition and should clear up in a week or so.*
  – *This is not a serious condition. These tablets should help.*

- Remember that **solutions** only work if they fit with the patient:

  – *Luckily enough, there is no need for immediate surgery.*
  Physiotherapy and medication are all you really need for the time being.

- Encourage patients to contribute to the **discussion**; to ask questions; to seek clarification; to express doubts, concerns and fears; and to indicate where they see a need for action:

  – *Is there anything you'd like to ask me?*
  – *Does that make sense?*
  – *This was quite complicated. Would you like to tell me what you think we have agreed?*

4.4.3 Negotiating the Management Plan

In the Western world of *patient-centred medicine*, effective explaining and planning the management aim not only for a shared understanding of the patient's course of treatment but also to have the patient share in the decision-making related to that management plan. When patients feel involved and responsible for their treatment or management plan, they may also be more motivated to cooperate and adhere to that plan.

Ideally, negotiation takes place between equals. However, this is generally not possible in a medical consultation, because only one of the parties (here, you) is an expert in the material being negotiated. Thus, to the extent possible, you should try to compensate for this inequality. As a medical expert, you can compensate for these inequalities in both knowledge and power by:

• Offering understandable, workable and acceptable management options
• Trying to make the patient feel recognised and understood

Sharing decision-making and responsibilities by negotiation is an ideal model. Because it is a process that may require more than one meeting with the patient, it is not possible under all circumstances—for example, if a patient needs an immediate procedure or intervention for a life-threatening condition, negotiating treatment is not appropriate. However, negotiating treatment is particularly important for situations involving:

• Major interventions
• Disease states with no immediate 'best' management option
• Problems that allow enough time for shared decision-making

The following are **three main strategies** for negotiating a management plan. As with other parts of explaining and planning, these strategies address both the content (what) and the way this content is communicated (how):

Step 1: Start from the known.
Step 2: Offer tailored, understandable alternatives.
Step 3: Select the 'best' option.

4.4.3.1 Start from the Known

• While offering and explaining the different options, start from what the patient already knows, thinks, feels and expects (see above).
• Do not start an explanation without knowing your patient's ideas, beliefs, concerns and expectations.

4.4.3.2 Offer Tailored, Understandable Alternatives

• Think about explaining as a kind of **teaching**: your goal is to help patients understand the situation so they can make a good choice.
• Share your own ideas, thought processes and dilemmas. In other words, **think aloud** (see above). Explain your findings, including your assessment of the seriousness of the condition, what is causing it and the expected short- and long-term consequences:

> – *I can't find anything seriously wrong with you, but ...*
> – *Well, the lab results show that ...*
> – *Your test results look very promising/good/somewhat disappointing ...*

Use understandable language: remember, the goal is to create shared understanding with the patient.
- **Structure** all explanations to keep them clear (see above):

> – *The first option is to try tablets. The other option is counselling.*

- Provide detailed, clear **information** about all the elements of the treatment or management options being discussed, including further investigations, interventions, medication and order of events:

> – *Because of these results, I'd suggest you to have some extra tests. The test will consist of ... and it will show us whether we need to ... You will need these forms to make an appointment with ...*

- Assess the options, discussing pros and cons.
- Discuss the **implications** of each option:

> – *We could prescribe you some tablets, but we might also get the same results by putting you on a diet.*
> – *I would like to advise you to give up smoking. It's really worth it. Following a heart attack it may double longevity.*

- Check with patients to make sure they have completely **understood** the options. If they are missing important information, provide additional information and/or clarification:

> – *Is there anything you'd like to ask me?*
> – *I don't know whether that makes sense?*
> – *This was quite complicated. Would you like to tell me what you think we have agreed?*
> – *Could you tell me how you would explain your condition to someone else?*

- Check with patients to see if each option you present is **viable**: Are they capable of following through with it? Do they have physical or psychological restrictions that make an option impossible? Would they be comfortable with this option?

    – *Is this a realistic option for you?*
    – *Is this option feasible?*

4.4.3.3 Negotiate a Mutually Acceptable Plan

The objective of negotiating a mutually acceptable plan should be to select the 'best' option.

- Make sure you have given enough specific information on the risks and benefits of each option to allow the patient to make an **informed choice**.
- Give patients the opportunity to formulate their own **opinion** on the basis of the pros and cons given for each option:

    – *Does this make sense? What do you think?*

- Offer **suggestions** and choices rather than directives:

Instead of saying:	**You could say …**
– *You must eat every 3 h.*	→ *The point is to prevent a completely empty stomach. You can do this by eating something every 3 h, like a sandwich.*

- Encourage patients to **contribute** their ideas and suggestions about their choices:

    – *I would like to know what you think about this 'best' option …*
    – *I would like to know if you have any suggestion about how to …*

- Ask patients about their beliefs, opinions, concerns, expectations, feelings and fears of effects (dimensions of the patient's perspective) as appropriate:

    – *I can see that this is hard for you …*
    – *When you say this, you seem sad/disappointed/angry. Are you?*

- Determine the patient's **preferences**:

  - *As I see it, ... is the most important conclusion of our talk so far.*
  - *So, in conclusion, ...*

- State your own position or preference regarding available options, and give the **rationale** for your position or opinion. Doing so may help your patient accept this position, because it helps them understand *why* you believe it is best:

  - *My preference goes to the first option, ...*
  - *It is my preference because ...*

- Reconcile your patient's **agenda** with yours. This may be difficult if you and the patient have different ideas about what is best. In reconciliation, it can be helpful to first think about what matters most for you and then think about what matters most for the patient. This can help you prioritise different considerations:

  - *I'm sure we'd all agree with that.*
  - *I can sense that you are opposed to that type of medication. Would you care to elaborate on why?*

- When you and the patient appear to have agreed on a management plan, check mutual understanding and **acceptance** of the explanation and the plan by:
  - Asking patient if they accept the plan.
  - Confirming with patient that the plan has addressed their concerns.
  - Asking for the patient's reactions to and concerns about the proposed plans.
  - Picking up and responding to cues. If you do not see the patient looking as if he accepts what you say, continue to negotiate. Watch for *nonverbal leakage*, which is a discrepancy between what patients say and their nonverbal behaviour. This can suggest patients may not be entirely comfortable with what they are saying. They might say: *Yes, I will try the tablets,* while breaking eye contact.

4.4.4 Enabling the Patient to Adhere to the Management Plan

Effective implementation of a management plan requires effectively **enabling** patients to manage all aspects of the plan, particularly those that they may consider potentially problematic.

The main strategies for enabling the patient to adhere to the management plan are:
- Encouraging involvement (Sect. 4.4.4.1)
- Removing obstacles (Sect. 4.4.4.2)
- Looking for support (Sect. 4.4.4.3)
- Agreeing on your and your patient's actions and responsibilities (Sect. 4.4.4.4)
- Agreeing on targets, monitoring and follow-up (Sect. 4.4.4.5)

One method which is widely used in psychotherapy to help patients overcome emotional or behavioural obstacles to the implementation of an agreed management plan is counselling. In Sect. 4.4.4.6 we will briefly illustrate this specific form of advising and coaching.

4.4.4.1 Encourage Involvement

Involvement helps patients feel responsible, can empower them and reinforce their ability to help themselves. Patients who feel more involved and are more likely to follow your advice:
- When the advice seems important to them
- When they believe your advice and trust you
- When they understand why they should follow the advice
- When they understand how to do what they are expected to do
- When they were involved in the decision to implement the management plan
- When they have promised to do necessary things
- When they have faith in you as their doctor, especially if they are convinced of your respect and appreciation and believe that they will be rewarded for their cooperation by still greater respect and appreciation.

4.4.4.2 Remove Obstacles

Sometimes there are obstacles that prevent or discourage patients from following through on management plans. Looking for these obstacles and doing what you can to remove them will help patients adhere to their treatment plans. Specifically:
- Check to be sure that incomplete **understanding** of the problem or the plan is not an obstacle to compliance. If it is, you can provide additional information or further explanation to clarify.
- Look for **practical** obstacles, which may be easier to circumvent.
- Make things as **easy** as possible for your patients. Patients are more willing to do things:
  - If there are fewer things to do
  - If things to do fit in with their existing lifestyle and practices (tailored)
  - If they have all the resources necessary
  - If they know exactly what to do in case circumstances change
- In difficult situations, like trying to change entrenched and unhealthy habits or patterns of behaviour, the best first step is to help patients **define** what changes they would like to make. Then, **reassure** patients that they are able to do it, and provide appropriate support. This approach is far more effective than blaming patients for 'bad' behaviour or convincing patients that such behaviour is their fault.
- Serious or persistent emotional and/or behavioural obstacles may require **counselling** (see Sect. 5.5).

4.4.4.3 Look for Support

Support can make difficult tasks feel much more **manageable**. To the extent that you can, try to help your patient find support in their individual life situations.

*   Ask patients about what support systems they have available.
*   Encourage or stimulate their use as appropriate.
*   Discuss other support that may be available (e.g., local support groups).
*   To the extent that you can, make things simple and easy.
*   Think of the patient's social context. Like most people, most patients are more likely to do things:
    *   If they can do it together with someone else
    *   If they know that someone is likely to check on them
    *   If the people with whom they live and work are willing to help them

4.4.4.4 Agree on Your and Patient's Actions and Responsibilities

It helps both you and the patient to be clear about who is responsible for what and who will do what. Having specific **agreements** about each person's actions and responsibilities can be encouraging and enabling:

> *   *I'll be in touch as soon as we get the test results.*
> *   *You will receive a letter about the follow-up appointment.*
> *   *Dr N will get in touch with me after your appointment with him to discuss the results.*
> *   *If you feel this stabbing pain again, please come to the emergency unit.*
> *   *OK, so we agreed that you will try to walk half an hour a day and you will keep record of how it goes.*

4.4.4.5 Agree on Targets, Monitoring and Follow-Up

Having specific targets, monitoring and follow-up agreements are equally encouraging and enabling:

> *   *If the medication does not improve your condition by the end of the course/the end of the week, you should return for some more tests.*
> *   *If you don't feel better within a week, I would like you to ask for an earlier follow-up visit.*

4.4.4.6 Counselling

The aim of counselling is to let patients form an opinion themselves. This usually involves giving them the opportunity to discuss their conflicting emotions and behaviours and to find and make the 'best' decisions themselves.

Counselling makes use of the **techniques** of active listening and appropriate verbal and nonverbal language discussed in Sect. 3.3, but also involves facilitating patients' forming opinions and making decisions. In short, you want to ask patients the basic questions you normally ask yourself when faced with a problem.

Ideally, counselling should ask patients questions in a way that effectively encourages them to think and decide for themselves. The goal is to have patients master their own opinions, so they can guide themselves instead of being guided by others. Counselling is by definition also a form of coaching.

When you are in a situation that involves counselling patients, you may benefit from the following strategies:

• **Try to clarify underexposed elements of the problem**
  – Ask the patient to explain or define unclear, vague or abstract language.
  – *'Think aloud'* or *paraphrase* what a person should think about to start to solve the problem:

> – *I understand that you need some alcohol to relax in the evening. I'm just thinking aloud. If you could relax in another way, you would probably need less alcohol. Are there perhaps different ways you can relax?*

  – Interpret or rephrase the patient's story from another perspective. This can help the patient see their own situation in a new way:

> – *I understand that you feel more and more exhausted after a day of uninterrupted work. Can you think of any way to introduce a break in your day?*

  – Add or draw out nuances. This can be another way to show the patient that their story has different sides to it:

> – *I understand that you are very angry about the delay of the operation, but I notice some relief in your voice too. Am I right in saying that you are afraid of the operation?*

  – Confront patients with their contradictions. Point out conflicting elements in the patient's ideas and feelings:

> – *I can sense that you are blaming your husband for his lack of interest in your complaints. But I also hear you saying that you want to be strong and don't want to be a burden for other people. I can imagine that this must be confusing for your husband.*

- **Provide explanations of concepts or ideas to increase understanding and insight**
  - Lack of insight in complex matters, processes, happenings or situations frequently contributes to misunderstandings. More insight requires more information to be put in place (context) as building blocks. Putting these 'building blocks' in place should ideally be done by the patients themselves, with the support of counselling.
  - In these situations, how you say something is as important as what you say (see *Appropriate Verbal Language* and *Appropriate Nonverbal Language* in Sect. 3.2 and Sect. 3.3). It is important that explanations do not sound judgmental and that they do not firmly direct or guide the patient. Again, the aim of counselling is to teach patients how to guide themselves, rather than be guided.
- **Encourage the patients to go on in their search for the best solution or decision**
  - Provide positive feedback: show respect and appreciation for the patient's efforts.
  - Help the patient reframe, giving a positive meaning to negative feelings or experiences:

> - *I understand you are really worried about your elderly parents, but you are doing a great job supporting them.*

  - Try using a stepwise approach to give the patient time to organise their ideas and not be overwhelmed:

> - *Perhaps it is indeed better to first make a decision about …*
> - *Later you can …*

  - Look for sources of support in patients' lives: suggest that the patient discusses their ideas with other people before they make a final decision.
  - Remind the patient that you are available for follow-up or further discussions and always make the next appointment before you close the consultation.

4.4.5 Structure and Content of Explaining and Planning

The content of diagnosis and management plan may be extensive and complex. What follows are outlines or **mental maps** to help you structure this part of the consultation. As discussed above, structuring the content in a logical sequence aids understanding and recall for the patient. It can also help you adapt and adjust more easily: knowing what information (in what sequence) you want to cover allows you to focus on how best to adapt to patients' individual needs.

In the following, we provide three outlines:
- Explaining a problem and its management
- Explaining a procedure
- Explaining a medication

4.4.5.1 Explaining a Problem and Its Management

Here, a 'problem' could be a hypothesis, test results, a follow-up result or a (full) diagnosis.

- **Introduce the Situation:**
  - Announce the problem.
    In the case of bad news, you can express your feelings in the following way:

> - *I'm sorry to have to tell you that …*
> - *… the treatment hasn't been successful …*

In case the news is contrary to the patient's expectations, you can say:

> - *I can't find anything seriously wrong with you, but I know you still feel bad.*

  - Emphasise its relevance for the patient:

> - *These test results are important as they explain your complaints.*

- **Explain the problem:**
  - What it is exactly? Why is it a problem? How serious is it?
  - What are the possible causes?
  - What is the expected outcome or prognosis? What are the short-term and long-term consequences?
- **Provide options to solve the problem** (management options):
  - Describe the patient's options and their implications.
  - Assess each option: What are the pros and cons to taking this course of action?
  - Negotiate the 'best' option and give room for patient feedback.
- **Discuss potential obstacles** to the implementation of the management plan:
  - Consider the patient's situation and think about what obstacles they could face.

- Agree on how to overcome or try to address these obstacles.
- Agree on how to enable the patient to adhere to the agreed plan of management.
- **Conclude/close the session:**
  - Announce the conclusion of the consultation (signposting) and give a summary of what has been agreed upon, stressing the importance of the matter for the patient.
  - Give patients the opportunity to provide feedback, as they may like to accentuate what is important to them, ask additional questions or add something.
  - Finally, explain to the patient what will happen next and/or what the next step for them to take is.

4.4.5.2 Outline: Explaining a Procedure
- **Introduce the situation:**
  - Announce the procedure.
  - Announce and emphasise the importance of the procedure.
- **Explain the context:**
  - Explain why the procedure is required.
  - What is the relation of the procedure to the management plan?
  - What can patients expect before, during and after this procedure?
- **Explain the procedure itself:**
  - What should the patient do to prepare for the procedure?
  - What does this procedure mean for the patient: hospital admission, time in a day clinic...?
  - The procedure itself:
    Where will it take place?
    When will it take place?
    How long will it take?
    Who will perform it?
    What will the patient experience: pain? Other discomfort?
    What follows the procedure?
    What does the patient have to do afterwards? (bed rest? physical therapy?)
- **Explain the (anticipated) results:**
  - When are which results known?
  - How will the patient be informed? What then?
  - What are the consequences if the patient does not undergo the procedure?
- **Explain side effects and after effects:**
  - What is involved in recovery and/or aftercare? How long does it take?
  - What immediate discomfort will patients experience? (is anaesthesia involved?)
  - What sort of discomfort can occur later during the recovery (wound healing)?
  - Which unwanted effect or complications can occur following the procedure? How likely are these effects, and how are they best managed?

- **Give patients specific instructions:**
  - Before the procedure (the preparation):
    When should they be present?
    Where should they be present?
    What should they bring with them?
    In what state should they arrive: fasting? …
  - During the procedure:
    What can the patient do or not do to facilitate the procedure?
  - Following the procedure:
    What will the patient have to deal with following the procedure?
    Which effects should the patient watch for?
    Which effects should the patient not need to worry about?
    Which side effects require contacting the regular (family) doctor?
    Which side effects require contacting a member of the hospital staff?
    Which side effects require immediate, emergency care or attention?
- **Conclude/close:**
  - Announce the conclusion of this explanation. You can do this while stating (signposting) that you will give the patient other sources of information.
  - Give or refer to other information sources, explaining why and how they are useful:
    Leaflets or pamphlets
    Patients' association: meeting times and/or website
    Other sources of electronic information or support
  - Give clear and concrete information about follow-up appointments:
    Is there a follow-up appointment needed or only on patient's initiative?
    Is the purpose of the follow-up appointment a specific post-procedural investigation?
    Is the purpose of a follow-up appointment to explain results and create a further management plan?
  - Allow time for patient reflection and feedback.
  - Conclude your explanation while explaining what will happen next.

4.4.5.3 Outline: Explaining a Medication
- **Introduce the type of drug and how it works:**
  - Name of the drug: use the name on the packaging.
  - How it works: provide patients with the essence of how it works, avoiding excessive detail. Relate, if appropriate, how the drug works to its 'functional' name, for example, antibiotic and diuretic.
  - Make clear the aim of the treatment: cure, risk reduction or just treating symptoms?
- **Explain usage:**
  - How should the patient take the drug: swallow, apply a crème, etc.
  - When and how should the patient take the drug: before each meal? Without or without food?
  - What is the usual dosage: three times a day? …
  - How should the patient store the medication: in the refrigerator? …

- **Review possible problems:**
  - Are there contraindications?
  - What are possible disadvantages and side effects of this medication?
  - Does taking this medication create practical issues or potential problems (often related to side effects), such as driving? ...
  - What are the consequences of non-adherence?
  - What should the patient do if they cannot or do not take the drug in time?
  - Can this drug be taken with other drugs simultaneously?
  - Can it be used if the patient is otherwise ill?
  - Can it be used if the patient is or becomes pregnant?
  - When should the patient stop taking the drug? Are there a set of symptoms that indicate this?
  - When should the patient consult a general practitioner?
  - When should the patient go immediately to the hospital emergency room?
  - When should the patient call immediately for an ambulance to the hospital?
- **Conclude/close:**
  - Check the patients' understanding of the information you have provided.
  - Check if patient will be able to follow all the instructions.
  - Offer written information when possible, as appropriate.
  - Give patients the opportunity to ask questions.
  - If appropriate, set up a follow-up appointment.

4.5   Closing the Session

Closing the session is a three-step process that consists of:
1. Forward planning
2. Providing a point of closure
3. Saying goodbye
Communication problems at the closing of a consultation are not uncommon. If doctors and patients have different goals or agendas at this stage in the consultation—for example, if a doctor wants to close the consultation, while a patient wants further clarification of an explanation—can lead to conflict and frustration. Additionally, the end of the consultation may also be a point where patients bring up new and potentially major problems that have not been discussed at all. This is called the **'doorknob phenomenon'.** While this cannot always be avoided, having good communication throughout the consultation can make closing the session go more smoothly and make the doorknob phenomenon less likely.

The most useful **active listening skills** in the closing phase of the consultation are:
- *Summarising* the plans that have been made
- *Clarifying* the next steps for both doctor and patient (see *contracting*, Sect. 4.5.1)
- *Checking* that the patient agrees with the follow-up arrangement
If faced with a doorknob phenomenon, respond positively and offer to schedule a new appointment with the patient as soon as your schedule allows. It is best to keep

your attitude open, **collaborative** and **patient-centred** and reassure the patient that this additional issue is not an emergency and that you would be happy to talk to them further about it at another point in time. However, you may also be firm in telling the patient that their consultation time is, unfortunately, over.

4.5.1 Forward Planning

Forward planning naturally signals the closing of the session. Generally, forward planning consists of two tasks: contracting and safety netting.

- **Contracting** consists of agreeing on next steps to be taken by both you and the patient. Contracting allows each of you to identify your roles and responsibilities going forward.
  - When clarifying the next steps to be taken:
    Check whether both of you have understood the management plan correctly.
    Check whether the patient wants to add anything.
  - If patients are waiting on results of tests, state explicitly how the patient will be informed of these results and what they should do in the meantime.
  - Make an appointment for a follow-up visit or inform the patient when, why and how to follow up with you.
  - Acknowledge the patient and the good communication you have had, so that the patient feels respected and the communication channel is kept open.
- **Safety netting:** When the next steps are clear to all involved, it can also be helpful to provide information about what to do if and when something goes wrong. Here, it can be helpful to address some possible worst-case scenarios, explain to the patients what to do if things do not go according to plan and when and how they should contact you (or someone else), if needed. This 'safety net' is important because it reassures patients, helps them manage uncertainty and helps them avoid being caught by unexpected developments.
  When 'safety netting', it is important to include:
  - What the patient should do if the plan is not working.
  - What the patient should do in a worst-case scenario.
  - When (for which symptoms, which signs), where and how the patient should seek help.

4.5.2 Providing a Point of Closure

An end summary followed by final checking creates an appropriate, final point of closure for the consultation. Generally, it is best to first focus on the end summary, then clarify the management plan and finish by asking a patient to confirm that they understand and agree.

In sequence:

- **Summarise** the session for the last time. It may be helpful to ask the patient to provide the summary to be sure that they have understood what you have agreed upon. This is especially important if you suspect any kind of misunderstanding:

> – *Could you please summarise what we have agreed to?*
> – *Could you summarise this as you would explain it to your partner?*

- **Clarify** the plan of care as necessary to complete this summary:

> – *I'll be in touch as soon as we get the test results.*
> – *You will receive a letter about the follow-up appointment.*
> – *I will send a letter to the specialist explaining the problem later today.*
> – *If there is anything unusual in the test results, the nurse will phone you before your next appointment.*

- Leave the patient 'space to respond' and confirm their **understanding**:

> – *Does this summarise what we discussed?*
> – *Do you have anything to add?*

4.5.3   Saying Goodbye

Saying goodbye comes naturally after the main points of the consultation have been summarised and you have ensured that there is mutual understanding between yourself and the patient. If a patient seems to be reluctant to leave, you can also try closing the patient's notes (written or on the computer screen) and/or standing up and moving towards the door.

Sometimes it can be useful to put aside some extra time for an informal chat at the end of the consultation. Patients often want to share something personal at this stage of the consultation. If these additional comments suggest a new medical problem that requires additional attention (see the '*doorknob*' phenomenon, Sect. 4.5), let the patient know that you have understood and that you will make a new appointment to discuss what has just come up.

Additional Reading

→ Cross Cultural Health

Hall P, Keely E, Dojeiji S, Byszewski A, Marks M (2004) Communication skills, cultural challenges and individual support: challenges of international medical graduates in a Canadian healthcare environment. Med Teach 26:12–125

Hornberger K, Itakura H, Wilson SR (1997) Bridging language and cultural barriers between physicians and patients. Public Health Rep 112(5):410–417

Jæger K (2012) Adopting a critical intercultural communication approach to understanding health professionals' encounter with ethnic minority patients. J Intercult Commun August 2012:1404–1634

Mignone J, Bartlett J, O'Neil J, Orchard T (2007) Best practices in intercultural health: five case studies in Latin America. J Ethnobiol Ethnomed 3:31

→ Empathy

Buller MK, Buller DB (1987) Physicians' communication style and patient satisfaction. J Health Soc Behav 28:375–388

Ferguson WJ, Candib LM (2002) Culture, language, and doctor-patient relationship. Fam Med 34(5):353–361

References

Bickley LS (2007) Bates' pocket guide to physical examination and history taking. Lippincott Williams & Wilkins, Philadelphia

Bickley LS, Szilagiy PG (2007) Bates' guide to physical examination and history taking. Lippincott Williams & Wilkins, Philadelphia

Bonvicini KA, Perlin MJ, Bylund CL, Carroll G, Rouse RA, Goldstein MG (2009) Impact of communication training on physician expression of empathy in patient encounters. Patient Educ Couns 75:3–10

Chugh U, Agger-Gupta N, Dillmann E, Fisher D, Gronnerud P, Kulig JC, Kurtz S, Stenhouse A (1994) The case for culturally sensitive healthcare: a comparative study of health beliefs related to culture in six North-East Calgary communities. Citizenship and Heritage Secretariat, Calgary

Giles H, Gasiorek J (2012) Parameters of non-accommodation: refining and elaborating communication accommodation theory. In: Forgas J, László J, Orsolya V (eds) Social cognition and communication. Psychology Press, New York

Kai J (2003) Ethnicity, health and primary care. Oxford University Press, Oxford

Kurtz S, Silverman J, Benson J, Draper J (2003) Marrying content and process in clinical method teaching: enhancing the Calgary-Cambridge guides. Acad Med 78(8):802–809

Kurtz S, Silverman J, Draper J (2006) Teaching and learning communication skills in medicine. Radcliffe Publishing, Oxford

Makoul G, Zick A, Green M (2007) An evidence-based perspective on greetings in medical encounters. Arch Intern Med 167:1172–1176

Maynard DW, Hudak PL (2008) Small talk, high stakes: interactional disattentiveness in the context of prosocial doctor-patient interaction. Lang Soc 37:661–688

Pendleton D (1983) Doctor-patient communication: a review. In: Pendleton D, Hasler J (eds) Doctor-patient communication. Academic, London

Pendleton D, Schofield T, Tate P, Havelock P (2007) The new consultation: developing doctor-patient communication. Oxford University Press, Oxford

Prabhu FR, Bickley LS (2007) Case studies to accompany Bates' guide to physical examination and history taking. Lippincott Williams & Wilkins, Philadelphia

Schouten BC, Meeuwesen L (2006) Cultural differences in medical communication: a review of the literature. Patient Educ Couns 64(1–3):21–34

Silverman JD, Kurtz SM, Draper J (2006) Skills for communicating with patients. Radcliffe Publishing, Oxford/San Francisco

Tate P (2007) The doctor's communication handbook. Radcliffe Publishing, Oxford

Special Challenges in Medical Communication

5

In this chapter we will look at some special challenges you face in medical communication and care. These are not challenges in terms of the grammar or vocabulary of any specific language you use. They concern certain communication difficulties you encounter and outline ways to communicate out of your difficulties.

Contents

What to Expect in This Chapter
In consultations, you sometimes have to deal with challenging situations. This chapter focuses on four types of challenges. Specifically, we discuss challenges related to:
- The state of the patient
- The content to be explored or explained
- The communication channel
- Other tensions in the consultation

In this chapter, we will first discuss general strategies and skills for dealing with challenging situations. Then we will discuss how to apply these strategies in a number of specific situations you are likely to encounter. All of these skills will help you be a better and more effective communicator in your clinical work.

5.1   General Strategies for Challenging Situations

In your clinical work, you are likely to encounter many different challenges (Wiseman 1995). In some cases, it will be the patients' behaviour: some **patients** may be silent or difficult to engage, while others may be overly talkative or highly emotional. In other cases, the **content** of the situation may be challenging: in clinical encounters, you sometimes have to address uncomfortable or taboo subjects, such as death. Finally, sometimes the **channel** of communication creates additional challenges: talking over the phone or through an interpreter is often more difficult than speaking face-to-face.

Challenging situations require care and attention, but the communication strategies and skills you use are essentially the same as those you use in other situations (see Chap. 3 for an overview). However, when faced with challenges, you may have to be more aware of your and your patient's behaviour and communication and use the skills you have more consciously or deliberately.

In all types of challenging situations, the following are good general communication strategies:
- Listen attentively to the patient while keeping the interaction going.
- Try to clarify the concerns of the patient.
- Try to identify whether more than one issue is involved (e.g. both misinterpretation and discussing a taboo topic).
- Whenever possible, avoid additional disturbances such as:
  - Being in a hurry
  - Being interrupted by the telephone or someone entering the room

In what follows, we provide strategies and suggestions for the challenges of specific situations.

5.2   Challenging Patients

Many of the challenges you encounter may be related to patients' **mental or physical** state. Often, it can be problematic when patients are:

- Silent or very talkative (Sects. 5.2.1 and 5.2.2)
- Confused, in altered states or highly emotional (Sects. 5.2.3, 5.2.4 and 5.2.5)
- Angry or aggressive (Sects. 5.2.6 and 5.2.7)
- Older and possibly hearing- or vision-impaired (Sects. 5.2.8, 5.2.9, 5.2.10)
- Developmentally delayed or of limited intelligence (Sect. 5.2.11)
- Children with their parents (Sect. 5.2.12)
- With family members (Sect. 5.2.13)
- Experiencing personal problems (Sect. 5.2.14)

5.2.1   Silent Patients

When faced with a patient who will not talk, try to understand why. There are different kinds of silence: 'normal' periods of silence are necessary to collect thoughts and to remember details. If patients are silent because they are thinking, it is often best to wait and allow them time to collect their thoughts. This will help both of you communicate better. However, some silences do not contribute to productive communication. When you encounter these, the following strategies may help you move forward:

- Encourage the patient to continue:

> – *You are quiet … What are you thinking about?*
> – *I sense you're tense. Would it help to talk about it?*

- If you suspect the patient may be depressed or have a related psychological problem, shift your focus to asking about symptoms of depression:

> – *I sense you may be depressed. Are you? … Could you tell me what you are feeling right now?*

- If you suspect that the silence may somehow be the patient's response to you, ask the patient about their silence:

> – *You seem very quiet. Have I said something that has upset you?*

5.2.2 Talkative Patients

When faced with patients who are extremely talkative, the following three-step process can be helpful:

1. Give the patients 5–10 min of talking time.
2. Listen attentively and try to find out what makes the patient talkative:
   - Is this their normal style of communicating?
   - Are they just expressing their concerns using more words than other patients, or is something else going on?
   - Are they anxious?
   - Do they have a psychological disorder that might be leading them to talk excessively, for example, *flight of ideas* (this is a type of language which is difficult to understand because it switches quickly from one unrelated idea to another)?
3. After they have been given time to talk, take charge of the conversation and focus on what seems to be most important to you and to the patient:

> – *This is very interesting, but let's return to the main problem …*
> – *I would like to hear more about that, but for now, given the short time at our disposal, I think we should focus on …*
> – *I am sorry that I have to interrupt you, but I need to find out more about …*
> – *You mentioned … Could you elaborate on it?*

5.2.3 Confused Patients

Some patients do not have a clear narrative (see Sect. 4.2.1.1) of their symptoms or problem. Such patients may not be consistent in what they report or may indicate that they have every symptom that you ask about. When faced with these patients, try to determine the **source** of this confusion:

- Is it language- or **communication-related**? Sometimes patients do not understand the meaning of a word or label for a symptom, and this may make confused and cause them to provide inconsistent information.
- Is the patient experiencing a **psychological or neurological disorder** that may be causing this behaviour (e.g. Alzheimer's)? If so, focus your attention on assessing the patient's mental status.

5.2.4 Patients with Altered States

Some patients present in states where their ability to communicate about their symptoms, understanding what you say and make decisions may be compromised by their condition or by other factors. Examples of this include patients with dementia, patients who are delirious from illness or patients under the influence of drugs that can affect their ability to function. When faced with these patients:

- Try to determine what kind of information the patient can understand and process. You may be able to discuss some things with the patient now but have to wait and discuss others later.
- If needed, find a surrogate decision-maker and/or advocate who can help the patient.

5.2.5 Emotional or Crying Patients

For some patients, visiting the doctor can be a very stressful or emotional experience. Some patients are better at controlling their emotions than others. When faced with a very emotional patient:

- Give the patient permission to cry by pausing in your examination and responding with **empathy** (and a tissue). This helps in two ways: first, the crying itself can be therapeutic to the patient. Second, your acceptance of their pain or distress can be helpful.
- Make a quiet, **comforting** remark:

> - *I'm glad that you got that out.*
> - *I can see that this is hard for you …*

5.2.6 Angry Patients

Some patients may express anger during the consultation. This anger may be directed at you, their situation or have no clear target. When faced with an angry patient:

- Allow the patient to express their anger.
- If a patient's anger is justified, acknowledge it and do what you can to address the source of their anger.
- Avoid becoming angry in return.
- Name and acknowledge the patients' feelings without agreeing with them:

> - *I understand that you felt frustrated by the computer crash, especially as it's the second time it has happened to you here.*

- If an angry patient becomes overtly aggressive, additional action may be necessary (see below).

5.2.7   Aggressive Patients

In some cases, patients may become physically aggressive. Aggression is more difficult to deal with since it is often irrational. When faced with an aggressive patient:
- Stay calm.
- Alert security, for everybody's safety.
- Avoid being confrontational, not only verbally but also nonverbally: use a calm tone of voice and maintain a relaxed posture.
- If it is safe to do so, suggest moving to another location.
- For additional suggestions, see *specific approaches for conflicts with patients* (Sect. 5.5).

5.2.8   Older Patients

Older patients should not be treated as 'elderly' (which often implies 'impaired') patients but rather as individuals in their own right (Giles and Gasiorek 2011). When faced with older patients:
- Be prepared to be patient and spend adequate time with them. Do not rush older patients.
- Allow the patient to set the pace of the conversation and consultation.
- Communicate genuine interest in older patients and their lives.
- During the agenda screening and agenda setting phases of the consultation, consider the possibility that some problems the older adult is experiencing may not be on the patient's agenda or need treatment at this point in time.
- Be aware that older adults may require additional and/or more thorough clarification, summarising and checking throughout the consultation.
- Be aware that older adults may require more structuring, chunking and signposting during the explaining and planning phase of the consultation.

5.2.9   Patients with Impaired Hearing

Some patients may have difficulty hearing. This is most common with older patients but can happen with patients of any age. When faced with patients with impaired hearing:
- Try to eliminate background noise.
- Determine if the patient hears better on one side. If so, seat yourself on the 'good' hearing side.
- Speak at normal volume and rate, and try to articulate clearly.
- To allow patients to lip-read, face patients directly and in good light. Do not cover your mouth and do not look down at papers.

- Check understanding regularly:

> - *Does that make sense?*
> - *Have I made it clear?*
> - *Could you please summarise what we have been talking about?*
> - *This was quite complicated. Would you like to tell me what you think we have agreed?*
> - *This hasn't been an easy topic. Are you sure you will be able to explain to your partner what we've arrived at today? Would you like to try to explain it to me?*
> - *Is there anything you'd like to ask me?*

- If needed, consider writing out instructions (or making drawings) and then check agreement and/or understanding.

5.2.10 Patients with Impaired Vision

When faced with patients with impaired vision:
- Start the session as you would with any other patient: shake the patient's hand and use appropriate verbal communication.
- Orient the patient to the surroundings (e.g. explain where the chairs are relative to the table).
- Report if anyone else is present or enters the room.
- Always verbalise what you will do or are doing. Speak normally.
- Adjust the light for patients with low vision. Ask the patient whether they want the light to be dimmer or brighter.

5.2.11 Patients with Developmental Delays or Limited Intelligence

When faced with patients with developmental delays and/or moderately **limited intelligence**:
- Try to assess patients' ability to function independently. Their level of schooling may help you understand this.
- If you are unsure about a patient's level of intelligence, do or request a mental status examination.

For patients with **severe** developmental delay:
- Always show interest in the patient, but turn to family or other caregivers for decisions about patient care.
- Avoid talking down to patients: treat them as individuals in their own right.

5.2.12 Children and Their Parents

Children have patient rights just as adults do. When faced with children (typically accompanied by a parent):
- Build **rapport** with everyone: greet and address both the child and the parents.
- Address children **directly** and treat them as you would an adult.
- Allow the children to decide who will tell the story (i.e. the child or the parent) and how involved their parent(s) will be.
- Be aware that preadolescents and teenagers may be very **self-conscious**.
- Summarise frequently, especially when your attention is moving back and forth between the child and the parents.
- When explaining, address everyone in the room and make your explanations understandable for everyone.
- When planning, involve everyone in **decision-making**. You could, for instance, address the child:

> – *It's great that you have understood everything so far. Is there anything you would like to ask me or your parents? Is this a decision you would like to think about/discuss with your parents?*
> – *I understand that you have a different view on this plan, and I appreciate your individual view, but …*

5.2.13 Patients in the Presence of Family, Relatives and Friends

In many cultures, involving family in the patient's treatment process is expected and essential. This is especially common in **collectivistic** cultures.

Individualism Versus Collectivism

Individualism–collectivism is one of the dimensions of cultural values described by the Dutch scholar Hofstede (2001). He suggested that different cultures have different values and that these result in different traits and different communicative behaviours.

In **individualistic** cultures, the individual is seen as more important than the group, and individual goals are given priority over group goals. People think of themselves first and foremost as independent individuals and expect to be addressed and treated as such. Generally, Sweden, Denmark, Finland, the United Kingdom and Germany are considered individualistic countries.

In **collectivistic** cultures, the group is seen as more important than the individual, and group goals are given priority over individual goals. People think of themselves first and foremost as members of groups (e.g. families). Generally, Italy, China, Iran, Iraq, Malaysia and Mexico are considered collectivistic countries.

When patients are accompanied by family members, they generally expect you not only to address them but also to address their (senior) family members. This is particularly important when you are discussing patients' diagnosis, treatment and possible complications in patient's care, because it is often the family that will be covering treatment costs. The involvement of the family is especially important when delivering bad news. In some cases, patients' relatives may request that patients not be fully informed about their diagnosis and prognosis.

This is a very important issue: failure to understand the involvement or role of a patient's family can potentially lead to problems with trust, dissatisfaction, stress, conflict and patient's non-compliance of care. It is also important to consider how this issue affects time: medical decisions may take longer if patients want or have to consult with family.

When faced with a situation where family involvement is likely and/or important:

- Consult with the patient separately to determine their wishes with respect to family involvement. Often, a private meeting is best for this.
- If the patient wishes, discuss medical decision-making and other issues in the presence of the family (in an arranged meeting).
- Provide ample time for the discussion:

> – As we agreed I will now summarise your problem and its management for both you and your family here …
> – In conclusion, for this new angina (chest pain) caused by new vessel narrowing balloon dilatation is possibly the best option. It can be scheduled for tomorrow, but first, do you have any more questions?

5.2.14 Patients with Personal Problems

Sometimes patients present with personal problems that fall outside the scope of your medical expertise. When faced with these patients:

- Do not engage directly in their personal problems, but limit yourself to listening and asking open-ended questions, such as those typically asked during counselling.
- Let the patient talk the problem through. **Guide** the discussion with questions like:
  - What kind of support is available to you for this?
  - Which approaches or solutions have you considered?
  - What are the pros and cons of each of them?
  - Who (else) have you discussed the problem with?

5.3 Challenging Content

In some situations, it is the content of the conversation that is most challenging. Challenging content is often emotionally charged, so addressing it involves not only dealing with the content itself but also the associated emotions. The following are

particular situations involving challenging content, with recommendations for how to deal with them:
- Emotions and pain (Sect. 5.3.1)
- Bad news (Sect. 5.3.2)
- Sensitive and taboo topics (Sect. 5.3.3)

5.3.1 Expressing Emotions and Pain

How emotions are expressed and evaluated depends on factors such as cultural background, education and personality. Closely related—and important to understanding patients' perspectives and narratives—people also differ in the extent to which they show or express pain. Some **cultures** value **stoicism**: people from these backgrounds are unlikely to express or draw attention to the pain they are experiencing unless it is very severe (and they cannot help but do so). In other cultures, it is more common and socially acceptable to show and express both pain and related emotions.

> **Emotions Versus Stoicism**
> People from Japan tend not to talk about their feelings, especially not with people they do not know well (Takahashi et al. 2002), whereas it is more common for Germans, Italians or French to express their emotions.
>   Patients from the Mediterranean region, Latin Europe and Latin America also tend to express more emotion, whereas patients from East and Southeast Asia and Nordic and Germanic Europe tend to be more stoic.

If doctors and patients (and/or nurses) have different norms or ideas about what a given level of emotion or expression about pain means, this has the potential to cause **problems or misunderstanding** during consultations and other interactions with patients. This can result in patients being labelled as 'hypochondriacs' or seen as 'putting up a brave face', when what is really going on is a cultural difference in norms for expressing pain.

> **Cultural Aspects of Emotions and Pain**
> In a German hospital, for instance, a nurse might think that an Arab man who is complaining all the time and in a very expressive way about his pain is snivelling or perhaps even a hypochondriac. On the other hand, nurses in a hospital in Latin America might not take the pains of a Norwegian patient seriously enough because he is trying to control himself and be brave and disciplined (Domenig 2007). The fact that patients coming from Southern countries tend to express their pain in a more expressive way than patients coming from Nordic countries even leads to the fact that German doctors sometimes use the term— not politically correct!—*mamma-mia-syndrome* to describe patients to their colleagues who are, in their opinion, acting up and exaggerating their pain.

When dealing with issues related to expressions of emotion and/or pain:
- Be aware of how patients react to your questions. If you have the impression that patients feel **uncomfortable** because you are asking questions about their feelings, explain to them why you are doing so and why their answer could be important for your diagnosis.
- Try not to judge patients who are more or less expressive than others. Rather, consider their behaviour as influenced by their (cultural) **identity and personality**, and respect it.
- Ask for **specifics** about what patients are experiencing (e.g. rating their pain on a scale from 1 to 10), because you can never be sure whether you are facing a patient who exaggerates or understates his pain, relative to your understanding of it.

5.3.2 Bad News

Having to deliver bad news occurs more frequently than desired by any doctor. Honesty is vitally important in this situation but needs to be balanced with sensitivity to the patient's emotions. Generally, the process of breaking bad news can be broken down into five stages:
- Preparing (Sect. 5.3.2.1)
- Explaining (Sect. 5.3.2.2)
- Providing support (Sect. 5.3.2.3)
- Planning (Sect. 5.3.2.4)
- Closing (Sect. 5.3.2.5)

5.3.2.1 Preparing to Deliver Bad News
When you know you will be delivering bad news to a patient:
- Find a quiet **room** where you can sit together undisturbed.
- Schedule enough (or extra) **time** for the discussion.
- Encourage the patient to bring a **partner**, relative, or friend.
- Think ahead of time about how to break the news as **briefly** as possible.
- Decide which information you want to **share** and which information you can give as answers to questions at a later stage.

5.3.2.2 Explaining Bad News
When delivering bad news:
- Focus on the **patient**, but take the other people present into consideration: if time allows and if the patient consents, see both the patient separately and everyone together.
- **Assess** what the patient knows and understands already or thinks, fears and hopes.
- When delivering the news, choose **words** that signal that difficult information is coming:

> – *I'm afraid that …*
> – *I'm sorry to have to tell you that the news isn't good.*
> – *I know this is not what you expected.*
> – *I'm sorry this comes as a shock to you.*
> – *At this stage there is very little we can do but make you as comfortable as possible.*
> – *I know this is bad news for you, but there is still a lot than we can do for you.*

- Start with only the basic information, but be **honest**. Don't minimise the seriousness of the matter.
- **Repeat** important points.

5.3.2.3 Providing Support

After delivering bad news, your first task is to provide (emotional) support:
- Allow patients time and space, and allow denial.
- Watch the patients' **reaction** to see how they are taking the news:
  - Do they seem to understand the seriousness of the situation?
  - Are they coping with the information?
- As patients react to the news, listen attentively, let patients express their emotions and acknowledge these emotions.
- As needed, **repeat** the bad news, supported with the same arguments. Avoid starting any discussion; only **rephrase** and provide corrected information as appropriate.
- While repeating, break information into understandable **chunks**, wait for a reaction and give patients time to reflect and to ask questions.
- If the patient asks questions, try to answer **truthfully**, keeping in mind that news takes time to sink in:

> – *I'm sorry if this wasn't the news you expected.*
> – *Please take your time (to process the information).*
> – *Can I get you anything: a glass of water perhaps?*
> – *Don't feel you have to talk/say something right now.*
> – *Take a minute to think about what it means to you.*
> – *Anything you feel right now is OK.*

5.3.2.4 Planning the Future

At the point where patients are ready:
- Discuss what is to happen next and provide a **plan**.
- Break down overwhelming feelings and fears into **manageable** concerns. This can facilitate coping with the immediate future.
- Identify **support systems** (such as the patient's relatives and friends), and offer to see or speak with them as appropriate:

> – *Is there anything I/we/the hospital can do for you?*
> – *Would you like to talk to someone besides me, maybe a grief counsellor?*
> – *Would you like help getting your affairs in order?*
> – *Would you like me to call someone for you?*
> – *Shall I call you a taxi? Shall I call your parents or partner?*

For patients coming from other cultures, you may want to consider the following question:

> – *Would you like me to talk to your husband or your family about your disease or should I just talk to you?*

- Communicate to the patient that you are their ally in dealing with their situation:

> – *We'll work on this together …*
> – *Feel free to call me if you need more information.*
> – *Remember you can talk to our counsellors anytime.*

5.3.2.5 Closing the Session

To conclude, once you have made plans for next steps:
- Schedule a **follow-up** appointment in the near future.
- Give patients your **contact** information so they can reach you by phone (or email).
- **Summarise** what has been said, and give patients the opportunity to respond.
- Conclude with **instructions** about what will happen next.
- Make clear to the patient that you are there to answer questions at any time.

This approach is also useful when delivering bad news to family members or friends, assuming that the patient knows and agrees to you bringing the news to the said family member or friend.

Cultural Differences in Breaking Bad News

Different cultures can have different **expectations** relating to bad news (Silverman et al. 2006; Tate 2010). Patients from some cultures (e.g. Russia) may not want to know the full extent of their diagnosis, particularly if it is terminal. Patients from such cultures want the doctor to encourage them and give them hope, not to tell them that they are going to die.

In some cultures, it is also customary for doctors to deliver bad news to family members instead of to patients themselves. In such cultures, it is generally the family that decides what they will or will not tell the patients.

5.3.3   Sensitive and Taboo Topics

A sensitive or taboo topic is a topic that people generally do not talk about or talk about only with close friends or family (for an introduction about how to broach sensitive topics, see Chap. 3). Common taboo topics include sex and sexual relationships (including incest, paedophilia, intermarriage), reproduction (abortion, infanticide), death and dying, food and eating (dietary laws) and bodily functions (menstrual cycles, defecation and urination) (Douglas 2002; Steiner 1999). Talking about these issues is often difficult for people, but, it can also be necessary during a medical consultation. The physical examination can also be a sensitive experience for some. The degree to which patients are willing to discuss sensitive topics differs from person to person and can depend on both cultural background and personality.

When dealing with sensitive or taboo topics, the following are good general strategies to ease possible tensions:
- **Apologise** if you see that the issue raised is sensitive.
- **Announce** that you are going to ask a question which may be sensitive and explain why you need to ask it.
- If you sense tension, **explain** that you did not mean to offend.

In the following sections we provide strategies and tips for specific situations involving sensitive topics.

5.3.3.1 Alcohol
- Consider asking about alcohol use following the history taking about coffee and smoking. This helps patients feel it is a 'normal' part of the medical examination.
- Ask open and descriptive questions:

> – *Can you tell me a bit about your use of alcohol?*
> – *What do you like to drink?*

- If you suspect a drinking problem, **screen** for it by asking the standard questions:

> – *Have you ever had a drinking problem?*
> – *When was your last drink?*
> – *Have you ever felt the need to cut down on drinking?*
> – *Have you ever been annoyed by criticism about your drinking?*
> – *Have you ever felt guilty about drinking?*
> – *Have you ever needed a drink first thing in the morning?*

5.3.3.2 Illicit Drugs

• Consider asking about illicit drugs following the history taking about caffeine, smoking and medication. This helps patients feel it is a 'normal' part of the medical examination.
• Ask open and descriptive questions:

> – *Have you ever used any drugs other than those for medical reasons?*

5.3.3.3 Sexual History

• Consider asking about sexual behaviour following history taking about genitourinary symptoms. This helps patients feel it is a 'normal' part of the medical examination.
• Provide a **rationale** as part of your introduction to the topic:

> – *To assess your risk of various diseases, I need to ask you some questions about your sexual health and practices.*

• Choose **descriptive** words that the patient understands and explain what you mean as appropriate. Avoid using vague wording or euphemisms:

> – *By intercourse, I mean when a man's penis is inserted into a woman's vagina.*

• How acceptable it is to talk about one's sexual life and sexual practices varies from culture to culture. Patients from some cultural backgrounds may be extremely reluctant to answer questions about their sexual history, particularly when the doctor and patient are different sexes (e.g. female patient and male doctor).

5.3.3.4 HIV and AIDS

HIV and AIDS is a very sensitive topic for most patients: not only is the disease itself difficult because of its prognosis, but talking about it can also involve discussions of other taboo topics such as sexual practices and drug use (see Sect. 5.3.3.2).

Telling patients they are HIV positive is a difficult and very **delicate** task. Patients are often shocked by the news and afraid that they will be rejected by their partners, family and friends. They will need your support and support from medical and nursing staff generally. When discussing HIV/AIDS:

• **Explain** to patients why you have to talk with them about HIV and why you need them to answer particular questions, such as those about their sexual practices.
• Take a **detailed** history of sexual activities, drug use, past illnesses, foreign travel and blood transfusions to get a clear understanding of the likelihood of the infection.
• Frame these questions carefully, using **non-judgmental** language (see Sect. 3.2).
• If you believe your patient should have an HIV test, give your patient **information** about the nature of the test; the medical, social and legal implications of the result; the risks of transmission; and what behaviour that might reduce these risks.

- **Tailor** the information to the individuals' needs, in terms of both content and language. Patients must be able to understand the information you provide in order to assess the risks and benefits of being tested.
- Watch your patients as you talk to them and try to determine if they feel **comfortable**. If they look uncomfortable, you can try to reassure them that they do not need to feel embarrassed and/or anything you can do to make them more comfortable. In some cases, patients may prefer to talk to a doctor of the same sex (e.g. a female patient talking to a female doctor).
- If the patient is extremely uncomfortable answering questions verbally, you can ask if they would prefer to fill out a **questionnaire** rather than discussing these questions face-to-face with you.
- Do not make **assumptions** about what your patients do or do not know about HIV based on their national or cultural background.
- Do not **patronise** patients: speak to them as independent, intelligent adults.

Communication, Race and HIV

A study about the communication of HIV care providers in California found that Black and Hispanic patients were more likely than White patients to report that an HIV care provider had talked with them about safer sex practices (Margolis et al. 2001; Marks et al. 2002). The study's authors suggest two explanations for this fact: first, that HIV care providers may be giving more attention to prevention in these ethnic groups because they are increasingly affected by the HIV/AIDS epidemic. Second, some providers may—mistakenly, as the study also found—believe that Whites are better informed and practise safer sex more often than Blacks or Hispanics.

5.3.3.5 Death and Dying

The ideas people have about death and dying can strongly influence their behaviour. It is important to treat them with respect.

Concepts of Death and Dying

Religion plays an important role in people's understanding and coping with death and dying, since all religions assume that death is not the complete end of existence (Sorajjakool et al. 2009). Because of this, sometimes, people will have religious thoughts when they are confronting death, even if they have never been religious before. Religion can be a great source of comfort to people. Some patients will want to practise special rituals like singing songs, praying and reading religious texts, which make it easier for them to cope with their situation. To the extent that you can, honour patients' desire to do this. After the patient has died, their religious preferences may also dictate how they want their body treated. Their and their families' preferences should be treated with respect.

When talking with patients about their **spiritual needs:**
- Ask, gently, if they believe a religious power can be helpful for understanding their needs, even though it is a private topic and a question to which a lot of people do not have a clear answer.
- Although you may not understand or share the beliefs of your patients, it is always good to let them talk about these topics if they want to.
- Put patients in contact with someone of their faith who they can talk with, if they desire.

When talking with patients about **end of life:**
- Explore patients' concerns and feelings.
- Ask specific questions about the patient's wishes about treatment at the end of life. This includes discussing what the patient wants to have done in the event of a cardiac or respiratory arrest. Be honest about the odds of success of resuscitation.
- Take a 'values history': try to identify what is important to the patient and makes life worth living for them, to help you understand at which point living would no longer be worthwhile.
- Demonstrate your commitment to staying with the patient throughout their illness.
- Assure the patient that relieving pain and taking care of their spiritual and physical needs will be a priority.
- Consider encouraging patients to designate a family member or friend as a health decision-maker, in the case that patients become unable to make these decisions themselves.

5.3.3.6 Mental Health
When you have to discuss mental health with patients:
- Start with direct but open questions:

> – *Have you ever had any problems with emotional or mental illness?*

- Move to more specific questions:

> – *Have you ever visited a counsellor or a psychotherapist?*

- For patients with depression or thought disorders, a careful history of their previous illness is essential.

5.3.3.7 Pregnancy and Delivery
Pregnancy is not an illness but is a condition that requires medical care and attention. Some of the issues surrounding pregnancy and delivery may be sensitive to international patients and their families, and not everyone may be comfortable talking about them with a male gynaecologist (Meadows et al. 2001). Pregnancy can also be an emotional period.

Intercultural Communication About Pregnancy and Delivery

A worldwide increase in migration of women has led to the 'feminisation of migration' (Domenig 2007). Therefore, gynaecology and midwifery (in or outside of institutions) are crucial fields for medical intercultural communication.

Most cultures have rituals, beliefs and general standards of behaviour relating to pregnancy and delivery (Hodes 1997). While some of these are shared across cultures, it is also important to be aware of potential differences. A woman who is influenced by Islamic traditions might, for example, not want to take the baby into her arms directly after birth but would want to wait until the baby has been washed. In many cultures, it is not common to feed the baby right after birth.

Many cultures also have beliefs about balancing elements, and of the warm–cold system, which are supposed to affect health. Women who believe in the warm–cold system often consider birth to be a cold condition. It is therefore rather frustrating for them to be offered cold food such as yoghurt or cold tea after they have given birth. Issues like this are why it is important to ask women about their wishes.

One should also be aware that it is not common in a lot of societies for the husband or partner to be present during birth. However, experiences with, for example, immigrant Turkish families have shown that younger migrant families may accept having the husband/partner present at birth if it is proposed to them.

When discussing issues related to pregnancy and delivery with patients:

- Inform patients of the role of the **gynaecologist**/midwife.
- Inform patients of the role of the **partner** during pregnancy and delivery.
- Inform (international) patients about the system of **midwifery** and also provide information in writing.
- Talk about **lactation** and, where possible, provide information in writing.
- When treating international patients during pregnancy or birth, it is important to ask them about **special wishes** (e.g. presence or absence of certain people), traditions (e.g. the warm–cold system) and/or other rituals (e.g. singing) that would help them to have a healthy pregnancy and birth.

International Study on Pregnancy

A study about Tamil women in Switzerland by Buchs (1998) found that pregnant Tamil women would have liked to be able to attend prenatal classes in their mother tongue and/or where other Tamil women are present.

The same study also showed that international women who just gave birth are very happy to share their hospital room with other women coming from their home country.

If there are prenatal classes held in foreign languages, inform your patients about them.

5.3.3.8 Contraception

Migration, Pregnancy and Contraception
An unwanted pregnancy can occur in situations of radical change, and migration is one example of this kind of situation. Women generally do not want to get pregnant during such a difficult situation or transition. However, it can be difficult to follow a consistent contraception regimen during periods of transition and change, and so conception can be more likely during these periods. Additionally, many women who trusted in attentive observation of their menstruation as a means of conception lose control of this, because the stress of migration can be significant distraction and may cause the disruption of normal menstrual cycles.

Migrants can also have difficulty accessing or navigating to the health system of the country they have immigrated to and therefore may not be well informed about their options for contraception. Migrants may also be suspicious of official centres including information centres, making them less likely to seek out medical care of this type.

Communication problems can be another barrier. If migrant women do not feel they have the skills to communicate adequately, they are unlikely to call the doctor or an information centre and/or make an appointment. Speaking at the telephone is often even more difficult for non-native speakers than is speaking in person.

Finally, how to finance contraception is also an important issue. Often, women stop using contraception because they simply cannot afford it.

In order to facilitate access to contraceptives for your patients:
- Ask people if they want to talk about their **options** for contraception.
- Provide the necessary **information** about contraception (spoken and in writing).
- Provide information, if possible, about ways to **finance** contraceptives.
- As needed, make use of a **cultural mediator**—an interpreter knowledgeable about the health and education systems in both migrants' new and old countries.

5.3.3.9 Family Violence
Family violence can be a taboo topic and should thus be approached with care and sensitivity. When talking with patients about family violence:
- Explain why you are introducing the topic, so give a **rationale**:

> – *Many women tell me that someone at home is sometimes hurting them. Has this ever happened to you?*

- Move gradually from general to **specific** questions.
- Move gradually from easier to more **difficult** questions.
- Ask parents about their approach to disciplining their children:

> – *What do you do when your baby doesn't stop crying?*

- When you suspect abuse, it is important that you find time to spend alone with the patient, to discuss these issues privately.

5.3.3.10 Torture and Trauma

Trauma is seen as a process which includes the phases before and after a specific traumatic event, as well as the sociopolitical and historical context around the event. Migrants may have experienced trauma before coming to their new countries, and it is important to be sensitive to this fact.

Torture is a related experience and can be a taboo topic often surrounded by silence. Torture can have lasting effects on a person's psychological and physiological well-being.

Patients who have experienced traumatic events—including but not limited to torture—may suffer from *posttraumatic stress disorder* (PTSD).

Studies on Trauma

One study of the multiple, painful consequences of war experiences examined coping among war-traumatised Bosnian refugees in Switzerland (Moser and Robertson 2005). These Bosnian refugees had experienced the loss of family members and other loved ones; feelings of helplessness and loss of control; social and economical dependence; difficult employment situations; structural restraints; and general increases in health stressors. These ongoing destabilising experiences dominated the daily life of the refugees. Resultant loneliness, poor health and stress and sorrow related to family and missing members of the family were important predictors of the posttraumatic stress disorders symptoms of the refugees. This study found that 69 % of refugees suffered from anxiety disorders, 68 % from depression, 37 % from posttraumatic stress disorders and 36 % from somatisations.

To help support traumatised patients throughout their healing process:
- When you meet patients, be aware that they could have had—or still have—a traumatic experience with lasting effects.
- When a patient indicates that they have been traumatised, take them seriously and **acknowledge** what they have been through. This is a symbolic act against treating these experiences as taboo.
- Advise patients to seek professional **support** from a psychotherapist or psychiatrist. If possible, recommend someone or set up the first meeting for them.

5.4   Challenging Communication Channels[1]

Communication is easiest when we have both verbal and nonverbal information available to us. However, when one of these communication channels is compromised, things can get more difficult, and we can experience problems getting our message across. In a medical context there are two main situations in which this happens: **telephone consultations** and communication through an **interpreter**. In telephone consultations, people have to rely on verbal information only, whereas in consultations where people rely entirely on the interpreter or cultural mediator, they do not have the original verbal channel available to them and instead only have access to it indirectly.

5.4.1   Telephone Consultations

Talking over the phone leaves people without nonverbal signals like body language, smiles and eye contact, which usually facilitate communication. Since a telephone conversation relies completely on verbal utterances and cues, the information exchanged verbally is all people have. Words are usually taken at face value, so it is important to pay attention to what you say to avoid miscommunication:
When engaging in a telephone consultation:

- Be **systematic** in covering all the issues raised.
- Use the same basic communication skills as you would in face-to-face consultations but with increased attention. These include:
  - Making sure that you are talking to the correct patient
  - Listening actively
  - Encouraging the patient to keep talking
  - Asking for detail
  - Asking appropriately focused questions
  - Signposting and summarising
  - Listening for cues from the patient
  - Demonstrating empathy
  - Providing opportunities to ask questions
  - Giving information in manageable chunks
  - Explicitly checking understanding
  - Offering options before trying to agree on the management plan
  - Sharing decision-making
  - Repeating and summarising the plan
  - Arranging follow-up
  - Making an audio recording of the consultation

Phrases to deal with potential communication issues in phone consultations:

[1] We are grateful to Elena Tomassini (S.S.M.L Fondazione Universitaria San Pellegrino) for adding some useful information to the section about the use of interpreters and cultural mediators.

> – *I'm sorry, but I'm answering your call from a mobile phone, so, I have no*
>   *immediate access to your electronic medical chart.*
> – *Could you put that in an email please?*
> – *Could you confirm this by email please?*
> – *I'm sorry I didn't quite catch that.*
> – *Could you speak a little more slowly, please?*
> – *Could you repeat that for me please?*
> – *May I ask you to spell that for me?*

5.4.2 Communicating with the Help of an Interpreter

In hospitals, a range of people can function as interpreters for medical communication (Rosenberg et al. 2007):

• The patient's relatives, such as husband/wife, child or sibling
• Bilingual health-care staff with the same linguistic background as the patient
• Professional (authorised) interpreters

Each of these channels or communication modes has pros and cons (Bernstein et al. 2002; Bolden 2000; Flores 2005; Flores et al. 2003). Relatives know the patients well, but they can sometimes be heavily involved in the patient's history and have their own agenda. Bilingual staff can be helpful, but it is important to be respectful of the time that interpreting takes and other professional tasks and commitments those staff members may have. Moreover, we have to take into account that they are not familiar with medical interpreters' code of conduct and lack formal training. They may misunderstand the patients, make mistakes and/or not be aware of the need for repetition or clarification, or they may be unaware of the high responsibility and importance of the role they are playing (see following example).

Emotional Involvement

Sometimes, using relatives as translators can be problematic because of their emotional involvement. The following tragic story from Domenig (2007) is one such example: a woman, 6 months pregnant, was taken to the hospital as an emergency case because there were complications with the pregnancy. Her husband was supposed to translate to the woman that her baby was not showing any signs of life anymore and that they had to induce labour. When the woman saw the dead baby, she started to cry and scream. The staff did not understand why the woman was as shocked as she seemed to be. They found out only later that the husband had not been able to tell his wife the truth. Instead, he had told her that after the premature birth, they would be transferred to the paediatric clinic to save the baby's life.

Authorised interpreters are neutral persons and a good alternative to direct interaction, though they might unfortunately not always be available; often, they have to be booked well in advance (Flores et al. 2008).

In any case, at the beginning of the encounter, inform all participants that the interpreter is going to translate whatever will be said and is not going to engage in any personal conversation with the doctor or the patient.

When using an **interpreter** (of any kind):

- Seat the interpreter next to the patient so the two have easy **eye contact** and can engage in nonverbal communication.
- If they do not already know each other, first allow interpreter and patient to introduce themselves and establish a **basic rapport**.
- Introduce the interpreter to the items you intend to cover in the consultation.
- Explain to the interpreter at the outset that you need a **translation** of everything that is said, not a summary.
- Ask the interpreter to alert you to and explain cultural differences; this will help you to develop your own intercultural **competence** and prevent any possible conflicts.
- Communicate—also nonverbally—directly to the **patient**, not the interpreter.
- Talk **slowly** and clearly, avoiding terminology, metaphors and idioms to the extent that you can. If they are absolutely necessary, explain them in a simple language.
- Help the interpreter by **outlining** your goals for each part of the consultation and/ or by explaining your plan for the consultation.
- Make your questions and explanations clear, short and simple. Focus on the most important data to communicate.
- Pick up the patient's verbal and nonverbal **cues** which can indicate lack of understanding, such as signs of stress, lack of eye contact, facial expressions, lack of interest and/or lack of attentiveness.
- Try to verify **understanding** by asking the patient—through the interpreter—to repeat what they have heard. Never ask the interpreter to tell you what the patient has understood.
- Make sure to **discuss** the main issues with your patient.
- If possible use pictures, schemes, cards or other visual aids for a better understanding.
- Be patient and accept that gathering and giving information take more time and may be less effective and satisfactory.

5.5 Conflicts in Medical Communication

A number of other problems may also make medical communication more difficult and lead to **conflict**. Doctors and patients can disagree at the **content level** about a medication, a treatment plan or a referral, among other things. These are generally misunderstandings or differences in opinions. These conflicts can usually be solved by explaining and clarifying the content about which there is a disagreement (see Makoni 1998).

At a higher level, doctors and patients can also disagree about each other's **involvement**: here, there may be conflict related to what the patient thinks a doctor should do and vice versa. Patients and doctors may also have disagreements at the **relational level**: here, points of disagreement relate to issues like collaboration and power (e.g. who gets the final say or whether patients feel their opinions are being heard and respected). Such conflicts at higher communication levels tend to have an emotional dimension and thus require extra care and attention in how they are dealt with.

5.5.1 Conflicts at the Content Level

When addressing conflicts with patients, the main strategy is to try to find a solution to the problem that forms the basis of the disagreement. This often requires a step-wise approach:

- First, try to **formulate** the basic problem briefly and clearly. Asking the following questions may help:

> – *What do we disagree about?*
> – *What do we have a difference in opinion about?*
> – *Which unexpected event was unacceptable for the patient?*

- Then, invite the patient to explain his point of view. **Listen attentively** and ask **clarifying** questions whenever appropriate. Check your understanding and **summarise** periodically:

> – *Let me check if I did understand this correctly …*
> – *Let me check my understanding of what you mean …*

- In turn, make the patient listen to you when you explain your point of view:
  - When speaking, restrict yourself to just the key points.
  - Pause frequently.
  - Allow questions to be asked.
  - Repeat if necessary.
  - Remain cool, calm and collected.
- Finally, find a satisfactory and acceptable **solution** for both you and the patient. Compromise as appropriate. Here, it can be helpful to focus on what is really important for you and for the patient: ideally, you want a solution that satisfies everyone's needs.

5.5.2 Conflicts at a Higher Level of Communication

When a conflict is situated at a higher level of communication, you have to temporarily leave the content level of communication and try to remove the higher level obstacles. This approach follows a three-step process:

- **Step 1: Listen and define the problem**
  - Listen actively, and observe when communication becomes problematic, troubled or highly emotional.
  - Ask yourself what could be causing the problem. Patients tend to fall back on emotions when they cannot rationally follow what is being said anymore.
  - Ask yourself what the patient is trying to achieve, and consider what you are trying to achieve.
- **Step 2: Get a grip on the conversation**
  - Having formulated a diagnosis of the conflict for yourself, you can now make clear to the patient that you first want to clear up some 'bigger' issues before discussing the content of the consultation any further.
  - This usually helps the patient to acknowledge that there is a problem.
  - Explain to the patient what you think the problem is, and agree on the way to address it. Emphasise that this is a joint problem and that both you and the patient are responsible for the further course of the conversation.
- **Step 3: Negotiate a solution**
  - First, the patient has to acknowledge and respect your role as a health professional. Then and only then can you try to agree on the way to address the problem and its possible solution.
  - Work together to find a way to address the higher level issue that is affecting communication.
  - Do not counter emotional objections with rational arguments if the emotional stakes remain too high; this will not move things forward.

Once the higher-level issues are resolved, you can then return to solving common content problems.

5.6 Summary

During their encounter with patients, doctors may have to deal with challenging situations. When dealing with challenging **patients**:

- Clearly and explicitly structure your talk.
- Explain every step you take.
- Do not talk down to your patient.
- Acknowledge the other people present.
  Take your time.

When dealing with challenging **content**:

- Apologise if you see that the issue raised is sensitive.
- Announce that you are going to ask a question which may be sensitive and explain why you need to ask it.
- If you sense tension, explain that you did not mean to offend.

- Ask for specifics about what patients are experiencing, because you can never be sure whether you are facing a patient who exaggerates or understates his pains.

When delivering **bad news**:

- Be honest, but balance it with sensitivity to the patient's emotions.

The process of breaking bad news can be broken down into five stages: preparing, explaining, providing support, planning and closing.

When dealing with challenging **channels**:

In **telephone** consultations, people have to rely on verbal information only.

- Be **systematic** in covering all the issues raised.
- Use the same basic communication skills as you would in face-to-face consultations but with increased attention.

In consultations where people rely entirely on the **interpreter** or cultural mediator, they do not have the original verbal content available to them and instead only have access to it indirectly. Authorised interpreters are neutral persons and a good alternative to direct interaction:

- At the beginning of the encounter, inform all participants that the interpreter is going to translate whatever will be said and is not going to engage in any personal conversation with the doctor or the patient.

When dealing with **tensions** occurring in the encounter:

- Try to find a solution to the problem that forms the basis of the disagreement.
- When a conflict is situated at a higher communication level, you have to temporarily leave the actual content level of communication and try to remove the higher level obstacles.

Additional Reading

→ Communicating Bad News

Gordon T (1995) Making the patient your partner: communication skills for doctors and other caregivers. Auburn House, Boston
Lown B (1999) The lost art of healing: practising compassion in medicine. Ballantine Books, New York

→ HIV and AIDS

Margolis AD, Wolitski RJ, Parsons JT, Gomez CA (2001) Are healthcare providers talking to HIV-seropositive patients about safer sex? Aids 15:2335–2338
Marks G, Richardson JL, Crepaz N, Stoyanoff S, Milam J, Kemper C, Larsen RA, Bolan R, Weismuller P, Hollander H, McCutchan A (2002) Are HIV care providers talking with patients about safer sex and disclosure? A multi-clinic assessment. Aids 16:1953–1957
Moss S, Williams OE, Hind CRK (1996) Counselling for an HIV test. Postgrad Med J 84–86

→ Interpreters

Bernstein J, Bernstein E, Dave E, Hardt E, James T, Linden J, Mitchell P, Oishi T, Safi C (2002) Trained medical interpreters in the emergency department: effects on services, subsequent charges, and follow-up. J Immigrant Health 4:171–176

Fernández EI (2010) Verbal and nonverbal concomitants of rapport in health care encounters: implications for interpreters. J Specialised Transl 14:216–228

Flores G (2005) The impact of medical interpreter services on the quality of healthcare: a systematic review. Med Care Res Rev 62(3):255–299

Green AR, Ngo-Metzger Q, Legedza ATR, Massagli MP, Phillips RS, Iezzoni LI (2005) Interpreter services, language concordance, and health care quality. Experience of Asian Americans with limited English proficiency. J Gen Intern Med 20(11):1050–1056

Hudelson P (2005) Improving patient-provider communication: insights from interpreters. Fam Practice 22(3):311–316

Ramirez D, Engel KG, Tang TS (2008) Language interpreter utilization in the emergency department setting: a clinical review. J Health Care Poor U 19(2):352–362

Rudvin M, Tomassini E (2008) Migration, ideology and the interpreter-mediator. The role of the language mediator in educational and medical settings in Italy. In: Garcés CV, Martin A (eds) Crossing borders in community interpreting: definitions and dilemmas. John Benjamins Publishing Company, Amsterdam, pp 245–266

→ Torture and Trauma

Basoglu M (ed) (1992) Torture and its consequences. Current treatment approaches. Cambridge University Press, Cambridge

Human D, Genefke I (1999) Torture and psychiatry. Challenges in the diagnosis and treatment of sequels to torture and extreme violence in the next century. Torture 9(3): 82–83

Wicker HR (2005) Traumatic neurosis, PTSD, and beyond: the rise and fall of a concept. In Department of Migration SRC (ed) In the aftermath of war and torture. Coping with long-term traumatization, suffering and loss. Seismo Verlag, Zürich, pp 149–170

References

Bernstein J, Bernstein E, Dave E, Hardt E, James T, Linden J, Mitchell P, Oishi T, Safi C (2002) Trained medical interpreters in the emergency department: effects on services, subsequent charges, and follow-up. J Immigr Health 4:171–176

Bolden G (2000) Towards understanding practices of medical interpreting: interpreters' involvement in history taking. Discourse Stud 2(4):387–419

Buchs K (1998) Tamilische Frauen in der Schweizer Geburtshilfe. Eine handlungsorientierte Studie zur Prävention pathologischer Schwangerschafts- und Geburtsverläufe mit Berücksichtigung kulturspezifischer Ressourcen. Arbeitsblätter Nr.17, Institut für Ethnologie, Universität Bern

Domenig D (ed) (2007) Transkulturelle Kompetenz: Lehrbuchbuch für Pflege-, Gesundheits- und Sozialberufe. Hans Huber, Bern

Douglas M (2002) Purity and danger: an analysis of concepts of pollution and taboo. Routledge, Oxford

Flores G (2005) The impact of medical interpreter services on the quality of health care: a systematic review. Med Care Res Rev 62(3):255–299

Flores G, Barton Laws M, Mayo SJ, Zuckerman B, Abreu M, Medlina L, Hardt EJ (2003) Errors in medical interpretation and their potential clinical consequences in pediatric encounters. Pediatrics 111(1):6–14

Flores G, Torres S, Holmes LJ, Salas-Lopez D, Youdelan MK, Tomany-Korman SC (2008) Access to hospital interpreter services for limited English proficient patients in New Jersey: a statewide evaluation. J Health Care Poor Underserved 19(2):391–415

Giles H, Gasiorek J (2011) Intergenerational communication practices. In: Schaie KW, Willis SL (eds) Handbook of the psychology of aging. Elsevier, New York, pp 231–245

Hodes RM (1997) Cross-cultural medicine and diverse health beliefs. Ethiopians Abroad. West J Med 166:29–36

Hofstede G (2001) Culture's consequences: comparing values, behaviors, institutions, and organizations across nations. Sage Publications, Thousand Oaks

Makoni S (1998) Conflict and control in intercultural communication: a case study of compliance-gaining strategies in interactions between black nurses and white residents in a nursing home in Cape Town, South Africa. Multilingua 17:227–248

Margolis AD, Wolitski RJ, Parsons JT, Gomez CA (2001) Are healthcare providers talking to HIV-seropositive patients about safer sex? Aids 15:2335–2338

Marks G, Richardson JL, Crepaz N, Stoyanoff S, Milam J, Kemper C, Larsen RA, Bolan R, Weismuller P, Hollander H, McCutchan A (2002) Are HIV care providers talking with patients about safer sex and disclosure? A multi-clinic assessment. Aids 16:1953–1957

Meadows L, Thurston WE, Melton C (2001) Immigrant women's health. Soc Sci Med 52:1451–1458

Moser C, Robertson E (2005) Bosnian refugees reconstructing their lives in the context of migration. An anthropological perspective on traumatization and coping processes. In: Department of Migration SRC (ed) In the aftermath of war and torture. Coping with long-term traumatization, suffering and loss. Seismo Verlag, Zürich, pp 17–74

Rosenberg E, Leanza Y, Seller R (2007) Doctor-patient communication in primary care with an interpreter: physician perceptions of professional and family interpreters. Patient Educ Couns 67:286–292

Silverman J, Kurtz S, Draper J (2006) Skills for communicating with patients. Radcliffe Publishing, Oxford/New York

Sorajjakool S, Carr MF, Nam J (2009) World religions for healthcare professionals. Routledge, New York

Steiner FB (1999) Taboo. Berghahn Books, Oxford

Takahashi KNO, Antonucci TC, Akiyama H (2002) Commonalities and differences in close relationships among the Americans and Japanese: a comparison by the individualism/collectivism concept. Int J Behav Dev 26(5):453–465

Tate P (2010) The doctor's communication handbook. Radcliffe Publishing, Oxford/New York

Wiseman RL (1995) Intercultural communication theory. Sage Publications, Thousand Oaks/London/New Delhi

Terminology

Medical Communication Skills: A Resource Book for Foreign and Mobile Medical Professionals

Acknowledging cues	Showing the patient that you have seen or heard what they are trying to communicate. Ways to do this include nodding or saying short phrases like 'uh huh' (Attentive listening)
Active listening	Listening in a way that is attentive to what speakers are saying and responsive to their messages. The first step to effective communication
Agenda screening	Checking with the patients that you have heard and understood everything that they wish to discuss
Agenda setting	Agreeing how to proceed next; naturally follows agenda screening
Appearance	How you look, including elements like the clothes you wear, your haircut and posture
Attentive listening	(Active listening) Listening in a way that is attentive to what speakers are saying and responsive to their messages. The first step to effective communication
Being healthy	A balance of physical, mental and social well-being, sometimes referred to as the 'health triangle'
Beneficent paternalism	Acting like well-meaning parents (how doctors often act when dealing with patients)
Biomedical agenda	The agenda you follow as a doctor during consultation
Body language	(Kinesics) The way you move, use your body and hold yourself (posture). This conveys a lot of information to others watching you

Building rapport	Developing a (professional) relationship between you and your interactants (patients and colleagues) through the way you communicate
Checking	Seeing if patients understand the information you have provided before moving on within or to the next chunk
Chunking	Breaking down long or complex explanations into digestible pieces
Chunking and checking	Breaking down long or complex explanations into digestible pieces and then making sure that patients have understood the information in one chunk before moving on to the next chunk
Clarification	Making things clearer. This is needed when statements are too vague or require further elaboration
Clear language	Using concrete words and phrases rather than vague or ambiguous words
Closed questions	Focused questions which require a focused answer, used to get specific and often important information (>< Focused medical history)
Complete medical history	A comprehensive history, covering all aspects of patient's background. This is the type of medical interview that medical students are generally taught to perform. This type of interview is also routinely done to complete hospital medical records (which may be a cooperative process between medical students and junior staff in academic and/or teaching hospitals)
Concerns	Worries and fears about the health problem, its implications and its effects on the patient's personal, family and occupational life
Consultation tasks	A doctor has five sequential major tasks to perform during a consultation: initiating the session, information gathering, the physical examination, explaining and planning and closing the session
Contracting	Agreeing on next steps to be taken by both you and the patient. This allows each of you to identify your roles and responsibilities going forward
Cues	Verbal and nonverbal signals by one person that are picked up by another
Directed questions	(Focused questions) Relatively open questions which allow you to ask for clarification or additional information

Disease	(>< Health) A pathological process, most often physical in nature (e.g. a throat infection). There is an element of objectivity about disease, because it is tangible: doctors are able to see, touch and measure it. In the dual track model, the doctor's track focuses on disease
Doctor's agenda	(>< Patient's agenda) The doctor's information gathering agenda, based on traditional medical history taking, guided by the patient's complaint(s)
Doorknob phenomenon	When patients bring up new and potentially major problems that have not been discussed at all at the very end of the consultation (just as your hand is on the doorknob)
Dual track model of consultation	(Two-agendas/two-perspectives model) A model of the consultation that addresses both the doctor's (biomedical) perspective and the patient's (illness) perspective
Echoing	(Repetition) Repeating (one of) the last few words of a patient's sentence when they pause to encourage them to keep talking
Egalitarian cultures	(>< Hierarchical cultures) Cultures that have relatively flat social hierarchies. Patients from egalitarian cultures, e.g. Sweden, expect to be treated more like a peer and see a doctor as an advisor. They want to be involved in discussions and decisions. They expect rationales and explanations and may question or challenge you and your suggestions
Empathy	Feeling *like* someone else feels. This may be difficult (and sometimes impossible) with some patients. You can however always try to understand their feelings. Try to put yourself in the patient's shoes. This may facilitate real empathy: thinking and feeling like the patient and understanding and feeling their perspective (their ideas, their concerns and their expectations)
End summary	(>< Internal summary or internal memory) A summary at the end of the information gathering, closing the consultation

Eye contact	Looking another person in the eye. This usually communicates interest and attention
Expectations	The information, the involvement and the care that patients expect, hope or wish for, and how they feel about these expectations
Explaining and planning	The second half of the consultation has two parts: (1) explaining the diagnosis and (2) agreeing on the management plan that follows from this diagnosis. Generally, arriving at a working management plan has two phases: (1) negotiating the plan and (2) implementing the plan
Explicit categorisation	Signposting statements explicitly naming all different chunks or categories, e.g. *I will now tell you what I think is wrong, then what I expect to happen and finally what can be done*
Explicit highlighting	Verbally drawing attention to a particular point
Face-to-face contact	Form of communication where both verbal and nonverbal information is available to speakers
First impressions	The initial 'picture' one person forms of another person. First impressions are powerful and can be difficult to change once they are established. A large part of first impressions are based on nonverbal, rather than verbal, behaviour
Focused medical history	(>< Complete medical history) The focused history is substantially shorter in duration and narrower in scope than a complete history. A focused history involves much more limited and closed questioning than a complete history
Focused questions	(Directed questions) Open questions which allow you to ask for clarification or additional information
Frame of reference	A perspective or way of seeing the world; it influences how patients think about their health problem, its causes, effects and management
Future-oriented cultures	(>< Present-oriented cultures) Cultures that focus on events in the future. Patients in more future-oriented cultures (e.g. Asian cultures) are generally more interested in preventive health care, such as regular check-ups, dental care, immunisation and screenings
Gap-filling	Small talk (e.g. talk about the weather) for situations in which you have to wait for some information or a procedure to start

Haptics	How touch is used in interaction with other people
Health	(>< Illness, disease, sickness)
	A state of physical, mental and social well-being and not merely the absence of disease or infirmity. A positive concept emphasising social and personal resources as well as physical capacities
Health triangle	A balance of physical, mental and social well-being
Hierarchical cultures	(>< Egalitarian cultures)
	A cultural with a clear and well-defined social hierarchy. Patients from more hierarchical cultures, e.g. China, may expect and/or prefer a more authoritarian style of interaction
Honest language	(Truthful language)
	Language that presents information truthfully; it is facilitated by clear (not vague or ambiguous) and descriptive (non-judgmental) language
ICE triad	(Ideas, concerns and expectations)
	Patients go to a doctor not with just a symptom but with ideas and concerns about their symptom(s) and with expectations related to their symptom(s). Feelings and emotions as well as the effects of the problem on their lives also play an important role
Ideas	What patients think and feel about their health problem, its causes, its effects and its management, (influenced by their health understanding or health beliefs) and about life and society in general (the patient's frame of reference)
Illness	(>< Health)
	The experience of feeling unhealthy. This is subjective and personal; it is a person's perception of their health, regardless of whether they in fact have a disease. In the dual track model, the patient's track focuses on illness
Internal summary	(Internal memory >< end summary)
	The summary the information gathered up to a given point in an interview. This is as opposed to 'end summary', which is a summary at the end of the information gathering
Kinesics	(Body language)
	The way you move and use your body
Listening	Good listening is active listening

Medical history	The complete medical history is comprehensive, covering all aspects of patient's background. The focused history is substantially shorter in duration and narrower in scope than complete histories. A focused history involves much more limited closed questioning than a complete history
Mental map	A plan of how the consultation will go
Meta-communication	Verbal communication about what is going to be discussed next: communication about communication
Metaphor	A figure of speech
Non-judgmental language	Words and terms that describe the problem at hand in a neutral way
Nonverbal behaviour	Everything a person does that is not spoken communication (verbal behaviour). In most cases, nonverbal behaviour will support verbal behaviour. If the two contradict each other, people tend to believe the nonverbal message more than the verbal message
Nonverbal communication	(Paralanguage) All elements of communication that are not spoken words. This includes the way we are dressed, the way we move, our tone of voice and our voice modulation and our use of silence. Our attitudes about what we say are often communicated through our nonverbal communication
Nonverbal encouragement	(One of the skills of active listening) Encouraging someone to continue speaking via nonverbal means such as eye contact, body posture and movement
Open questions	Broad questions giving patients freedom to choose how they respond
Open-to-closed cone of questioning	A strategy for gathering information starting with open questions, followed by focused questions and then closed questions
Paralanguage	Elements of nonverbal communication that relate to how we speak, including tone of voice and voice modulation
Paraphrasing	Restating in your own words what you have heard or understood

Patient narratives	The stories as told by patients in their own words about the problems they are experiencing. These are generally told chronologically from when the problem first started to the present. Patients' narratives are an important source of information about patients' medical issues, but how you handle them also affects patients' impressions of you and how much trust and confidence they place in you later
Patient-oriented medicine	An approach to medicine, common in the West, which considers not only the doctor's perspective but also the patient's
Patient's agenda	(>< Doctor's agenda) The patient's ideas, concerns and expectations with which they come to see you
Patient's illness perspective	(>< Doctor's disease perspective) The patient's agenda for the consultation which reflects the patient's perspective of the problem
Picking up cues	Observing and acknowledging cues in patients' verbal and nonverbal behaviour. Picking up on cues is one way to discover the patient's hidden agenda
Posture, proxemics and haptics	The use of body language
Present-oriented cultures	(>< Future-oriented cultures) Cultures that focus on events in the present. Patients in more present-oriented cultures (e.g. many African cultures) generally show less interest in preventative health care, such as regular check-ups, dental care, immunisations and screenings
Primacy effect	(>< Recency effect) Effect of selective memory that recalls best what was told first
Procedural safety net	(>< Relational safety net) The procedural 'safety net' involves knowing and understanding the examination or procedure you are carrying out and knowing what will come next
Providing rationale	(Sharing thoughts) Sharing the reasons for your actions and questions
Proxemics	Use of space and the distance you put between yourself and other people

Rapport	Developing a good relationship between people. This is done in part through communication
Recency effect	(>< Primacy effect) Effect of selective memory that recalls the latest information better
Recognisable language	Using words and phrases that the patient knows
Reflection of feelings	Summarising and playing back your impression of the feelings or emotions that others are experiencing. This is usually done with a short question or comment checking your interpretation of what patients are feeling
Relational safety net	(>< Procedural safety net) Reassuring patients that you are a professional and an expert and that you care for them and their well-being
Repetition	(Echoing) Repeating (one of) the last few words of a patient's sentence when they pause to encourage them to keep talking
Respectful language	Language that demonstrates respect and attention, uses descriptive (rather than judgmental) words and is problem-oriented (focused on the patient's medical issue)
Responding to cues	Acknowledging a cue and investigating what it means and what it can tell you about the patient's perspective, ideas, concerns and expectations
Safety netting	Providing information about what to do if and when something goes wrong. This 'safety net' is important because it reassures patients, helps them manage uncertainty and helps them avoid being caught by unexpected developments
Sharing thoughts	(Providing rationale) Sharing your reasons for your actions and questions
Sickness	(>< Health) The external and public mode of not being healthy. Sickness is a social role, a state, a negotiated position in the world: it can be thought of as an 'agreement' between the person henceforward called 'sick' and a society which is prepared to recognise him as such
Signposting	An explicit statement telling the patient what you are about to say or do (often a change of direction)

Silence	Not speaking. This can carry different meaning from person to person and from culture to culture
Simple language	Language that avoids jargon, abbreviations and complex words and phrases
Structuring	Sequencing actions in an ordered way (possibly making use of a mental map)
Summarising	Restating all of the important points in a discussion
Symptom analysis	The process of gathering more information about patients' symptoms, usually following a patient's narrative
Symptom dimensions	Different aspects of the symptoms patients describe. A mnemonic for *symptom dimensions* is *WWQQAA + B*: **W**hen (timing), **W**here (location), **Q**uality (character), **Q**uantity (severity), **A**ggravating (+setting) and alleviating factors (+therapy), **A**ssociated symptoms + **B**eliefs
Timing information	When information is provided. Research has shown that we remember information at the beginning and end of the conversations best, so these are the best times to provide important information
Tone and use of voice	How voice is used in conversation. This includes speed, articulation, modulation and volume. Tone of voice carries information about who we are. It is an important indicator of our level of interest, engagement and knowledge
Truthful language	(Honest language)
	Language that presents information truthfully, it is facilitated by clear (not vague or ambiguous) and descriptive (non-judgmental) language
Two-agendas consultation model	(Two-perspectives/dual track model)
	A model of the consultation that addresses both the doctor's (biomedical) perspective and the patient's (illness) perspective
Two-perspectives consultation model	(Two-agendas model)
	A model of the consultation that addresses both the doctor's (biomedical) perspective and the patient's (illness) perspective
Understandable language	Simple, recognisable and clear words and phrases to ask questions, explain and plan
Verbal communication	Spoken words. Appropriate verbal communication is understandable, respectful and honest

Verbal and nonverbal channels	Both channels should be used consistently. Otherwise, this may cause confusion and undermine other's trust and belief in your sincerity and honesty
Verbal encouragement	(One of the skills of active listening) Using short verbal phrases to show others that you are paying attention, acknowledging them and what they are saying (*I see, uh uh, ...*)

Index

K. Van de Poel et al., *Communication Skills for Foreign and Mobile Medical Professionals*,   143
DOI 10.1007/978-3-642-35112-9, © Springer-Verlag Berlin Heidelberg 2013